What *Are* People Saying About The Fat Burning Diet?

Dear Jay,

Congratulations on your book, The Fat Burning Diet! You offer many useful tips that will help a lot of people. I plan on implementing many of them myself. Best of luck to you in your endeavors!
—Denis Wilson, M.D., author of Wilson's Syndrome

I must thank you for The Fat Burning Diet, which has gotten my body looking better than ever! I used to eat a high-carbohydrate low-fat diet that kept me very plump! I've learned more from your fat burning book than any of the 50 books in my body-building library. Thank you, again!
—M.A. Hatfield, MA

The first week, I lost 4 pounds. My energy level stabilized, and I didn't feel hungry. The second week, I lost 3 more pounds. The third week, I lost another 2-3 pounds, and I was much stronger. After the first month on The Fat Burning Diet, I was down to 11.9% body fat!
—M.G., San Diego, CA

The first three months I followed The Fat Burning Diet, I lost 2% body fat each month—dropping from 15% down to 9%. I didn't increase my exercise level at all! After one year on your diet, my energy is so high it seems I can go forever. I engage in more activities that require a great deal of energy, yet I still feel like I can do more. I wish I would have known about your diet back in my high school and college athletic days. Thanks again, Jay!
—B.H., Liberty, MO

The Fat Burning Diet

I thoroughly enjoyed reading your book and agree with its phi-losophy. I have implemented your dietary suggestions with sev-eral of my patients and have seen great success. I continue to urge my patients to read your book. Thank you for your help. Best of luck.

—Edward J. Steel, D.C., C.C.S.P.
Steel Chiropractic & Sports Injury Center

I assumed, like millions of Americans, that a high-carbohydrate low-fat diet was the right one for me. After four years of regu-larly consuming high-carbohydrate foods and very little fat, my skin and hair looked like lizard and straw. I clung to the accept-ed belief that if I followed the advice of the health community and my doctor, I would eventually lose weight and my health would be restored. Unfortunately, I actually gained weight on my high-carbohydrate diet, and my cholesterol jumped way up. I was bloated, released gas all the time, had the energy level of dirt, and my feet and ankles were so swollen from fluid reten-tion that I couldn't put my shoes on.

Then I read your book and started following your diet. In the first six days, I lost 5 pounds of water and bloat, and my energy level skyrocketed. I no longer needed a nap every afternoon, and sleeping became a pleasurable night's rest instead of a wrestling match with my sheets. In just four short weeks, I lost 15 pounds!

I'm grateful to you for creating a diet that actually works. For a 51-year-old overweight housewife with Meniere's disease—a condition that prevents me from exercising—this revelation of fat burning secrets has been a godsend. I can't wait for your next book!

—K.C., San Diego, CA

Jay Robb
Certified Clinical Nutritionist

The
Fat Burning Diet
Accessing Unlimited Energy for a Lifetime

Loving Health Publications
in conjunction with

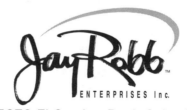

ENTERPRISES Inc.

5670 El Camino Real, Suite C
Carlsbad, CA 92008

www.JayRobb.com / 1.877.JAY.ROBB

The Fat Burning Diet

Robb, Jay
The Fat Burning Diet
Accessing Unlimited Energy for a Lifetime
Jay Robb

ISBN 0-9620608-3-6
1. Reducing diets. 2. Nutrition. 3. Diet—popular works.

Manufactured in the United States of America

Loving Health Publications
in conjuction with

Jay Robb Enterprises Inc.
5670 El Camino Real, Suite C
Carlsbad, CA 92008

Cover design by Eugene Epstein
Jay Robb's photo by Greg Aiken

Dedicated
to Our Creator

Thank you, God. When I was alive and well, You were always there for me. When I was down and out, You answered my prayers and gave me hope, direction, and The Fat Burning Diet so that I could regain my health. And when I was caught up in my ego and sinful ways of living, I asked Your son Jesus Christ to come into my heart and forgive me of my sins—and He did. I owe everything to You and have vowed to spend the rest of my life sharing Your divine diet secrets with the world. It is Your will, Your way...all the way! Thank you, Lord.

And a Very Special "Thank You"

—to my wife **Rosemary**. For each and every time I needed you to be there for me as a candid and supportive friend, you were. My love deepens for you with each passing day. Thank you for being my wife and best friend and for creating a beautiful spiritual atmosphere in our home and in our life. I love you!

—to my son **Angelo**, for *just being you*. Your spirit and joy shines bright daily, and that inspires me. The time we spend together will be treasured forever.

—to my mother **Joyce "Mamá" Roesing** and husband **Bill Roesing** for years of unfailing love, support, and encouragement.

—to my sister **Joy Graham** for *always* loving me unconditionally and supporting me through each phase of my life.

—to my sister **Jane Marie Mitchell** for being a shining example of how to walk strong with God. This has been a real blessing.

—to **Heather Aiken** for your hard work and dedication. Your desire to perform above and beyond by lending your expertise in editing has allowed me to create this book. You are awesome and truly guided by the Lord.

—to my entire staff at Jay Robb Enterprises Inc. Many thanks to each member of the "Jay-Team" for offering your never-ending support to keep the office and warehouse running smoothly and efficiently. Thank you (in alphabetical order) **Heather Aiken, Rick Cortez, Nancy Ferguson, Brian Giovannucci, Drew "FlashMaster" Goldstein, Joe Hernandez, Chris Martin, Julie Teuton, Reem Totry, Kathy Wolff,** and **Craig Zelent** for each and every contribution you have made to this organization. It is the combination of all of your god-given talents and time that has built, shaped, and made this company what it is.

—to my best friend **Bruce "Gobsapecs" Heflebower** for your unconditional friendship; to my good friends **Ron Cottingham, John "Abdoer" Abdo, Ken Davis, "Jimbo" Someck, Steve Downs, Luis "Luigi" Casillas, CJ Hunt, Guy Takayama,** and **Robert Harris**; and to my many friends at **KUSI Channel 9** in San Diego. Thank you for your consistent help and support.

—to **Greg Aiken** for your stellar photographic work which skillfully captured and created the Jay Robb image. Your ability to beautifully depict the essence of your subjects makes you an artist.

—to **Eugene Epstein** for your creative technical and design skills for creating this book cover. You are an extremely talented artist, and your contribution to this project is *truly* appreciated!

—to the **thousands of health food stores, gyms, nutrition and fitness centers, doctors' offices, and clinics across the nation** that carry our books and products. Your support is allowing us to reach and teach every man, woman, and child on this planet that desires to discover the health benefits of our glycogen-management program called "The Fat Burning Diet."

the fat burn·ing di·et: a time-proven revolutionary way of eating high-carb meals offset by low-carb meals to lose weight without the typical discomforts of dieting.

The author does not claim to be a doctor or healer of any sort. This book is intended for educational purposes only and should not be used as a guide for diagnosis and treatment of any disease. If you have any health problems, it is advisable to seek the advice of a health care professional of your choice.

A Special Note to You

However this book got into your hands, consider it providential—not coincidental. The material you are about to read was given to me at a time when I desperately needed a solution to my failing health. God, through His mercy and grace, gave me my life back—a healthier one that could be used to help, motivate, and educate others.

This book is your new roadmap to better health, a better body, and a more balanced life. God bless you on your new fat burning journey!

Table of Contents

Important Foreword from the Author about this All-New Revised Edition

After carefully listening to the feedback of thousands of readers and clients since 1980, I have intellectually and prayerfully considered every suggestion—which recently led me to update and revise *The Fat Burning Diet*. Now, *easier than ever to follow and understand*, this revision teaches the foundational principles of glycogen management—carb-depletion and carb-loading—but does so in a way that an individual who has no background in diet and nutrition can follow it and experience dietary success for a lifetime. The knowledge needed to create this manuscript I credit entirely to God—who worked *through me* from the creation of the program through the entire rewriting process.

What's New in *this* Edition:
1. New low-carb and high-carb meal cycles.
2. Menus and meal plans that are easier to follow.
3. A new heart-healthy supplement combination.
4. A clearer understanding of glycogen management.
5. New techniques for bodybuilders to get in contest shape.
6. More "dining out" ideas to make dieting easier than ever.
7. New ways to carb-deplete and carb-load.
8. A new way of eating less often yet feeling more satisfied.

Thank you for reading this all-new 2004 revised and expanded edition of *The Fat Burning Diet*. I honestly feel it is the best diet on the planet. I pray it brings you the health and well-being that God has planned for you.

> "Pride should only be associated
> with a pack of lions."
> —The Author

Introduction

She whispers, "For $50 I'll do *anything* you desire."

A man strolled into his favorite drinking establishment, settled onto a vacant bar stool, and ordered an ice-cold brew. Within moments, the man was approached by an attractive young woman wearing a very revealing outfit. Portraying sensual body language, this breathtaking beauty leaned forward and whispered in the man's ear, "For $50 I'll do *anything* you desire, but you must tell me your desire in three words or less."

Having just stormed out of the house—after a disagreement with his wife—the man's ears perked up a bit. Self-control and discipline outweighed the tempting request, however, and the man remained quiet, staring straight ahead at his beer.

Again, the temptress leaned forward and whispered softly in his ear, "For $50 I'll do *anything* you desire, but you must tell me your desire in three words or less." The man's ears now started to twitch as these soft words aroused a tingling in his body. Once again, his masterful ability to stay self-controlled stopped him from moving an inch.

Sensing the man's resistance was weakening, the tempting female goddess leaned forward again, this time purposefully brushing her soft upper body against his left shoulder. She whispered this provocative offer in his ear one more time, "For $50 I'll do *anything* you desire, but you must tell me your desire in three words or less."

That was it! The man's resistance crumbled as he realized this offer was simply too good to let pass by. Quickly rising from his bar stool, the man slid a $50 bill into her awaiting palm, leaned forward, and whispered softly in *her* ear, "Paint my house."

The Fat Burning Diet

Burn, Baby, Burn!

Every day of your life, you make choices. From the moment you wake up to the moment you go to bed, you make decisions that shape the direction of each day and, ultimately, your life. Past and present marketing data suggests that we, as a nation, are heavily influenced by the messages and images we're exposed to on a daily basis—consciously *and* subconsciously. It takes discipline to consider the realm of possibilities that would best serve our needs, as the previous story illustrates. The Fat Burning Diet is a way of eating and thinking outside the box— or should I say "outside the lunch box"?

Most Americans have no idea that it is easier to burn fat by eating properly than by exercising. In fact, what people eat actually determines if their body will be able to burn fat—whether they are exercising or not. The problem is that most Americans do not know what foods enable their body to burn fat.

The majority of popular diets on the market are either too extreme or very difficult to follow. Some diet gurus claim ALL carbs can make you fat and urge people to avoid them like the plague. Other experts claim that fat is the enemy and advocate the low-fat high-carbohydrate diet as a means of melting away unwanted fat and keeping it off.

The truth is: High-carb diets *and* low-carb diets work—but not *all the time*, as you will discover in the pages that follow.

FASCINATING FACT:
The secret to permanent weight loss is offsetting high-carb meals with low-carb meals. When you do this, you get what I call "The Fat Burning Diet."

In 1990 I shocked the world—especially the fitness world— when I nationally attacked carbohydrates and suggested that Americans limit their intake of carbohydrate and increase their intake of protein and healthy fats. When I started conducting seminars, I was the only one waving a "carb-control" flag. However, within five years after the creation of The Fat Burning Diet and the circulation of several best-selling books written by authors who agreed with my stance, our great nation saw a need to put the brakes on heavy carbohydrate consumption.

Because the nation had become so addicted to carbohydrate foods, in 1990 I felt it appropriate to attack carbohydrates and to present carbs as "the bad guys"—or my words would have fallen on deaf ears. The spark I started back then has now ignited into a full-blown war against carbs. Everywhere you go, you see labels that promote "low-carb" this and "low-carb" that. Our nation has fallen into a trap and has become carbophobic!

Ironically, many years later—since I first introduced The Fat Burning Diet—I now find it CRITICAL to teach Americans that carbs are *actually not* the bad guys and that, with discretion, they need to integrate them into their diet. I teach people the difference between good and bad carbs (carbs to avoid routinely) and how to ensure these good carbs will perform optimally. The secret is to limit carbs (not eliminate them) by simply eating high-carb meals that offset low-carb meals. That has always been the secret of The Fat Burning Diet and is what clearly separates it from other diets. When you properly offset high-carb meals with low-carb meals, your body can become an energized fat-melting machine.

This latest revised edition reflects 25 years of research on diet-induced fat burning and introduces my new revolutionary "low-carb high-carb" eating pattern for burning fat. I have simplified it so that anyone—regardless of what *shape* a person is in—can start the program immediately and maintain it for life.

God bless you on your journey!

Jay Robb

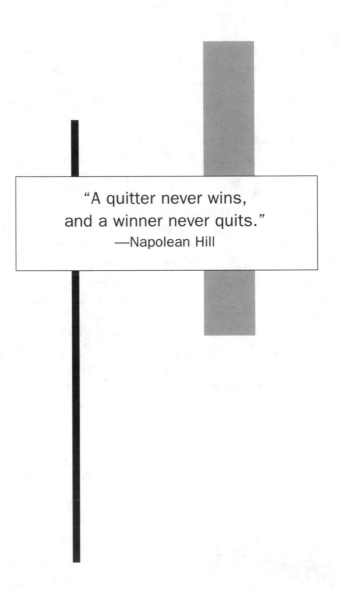

"A quitter never wins,
and a winner never quits."
—Napolean Hill

An Opening Prayer for You:

I pray that you will allow the words in this book to guide you on a journey to better eating and better living. I pray that you trust God, fully knowing that He *will* supply you with the strength, confidence, and courage you need to make this commitment for a lifetime. I pray that you will *never* take your eyes off the Lord but, instead, will follow Him and rely on His infinite power and wisdom. Lastly, my friend, I pray that you will take your hands *off* the wheel of life and let God do the driving.

—Amen...and enjoy the ride!

"I skate where the puck is going to
be, not where it has been."
—Wayne Gretzky

About
Jay Robb

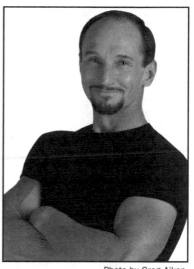

Photo by Greg Aiken

Jay Robb was born June 15, 1953. He is a certified clinical nutritionist with nearly 25 years' experience as a professional in his field. He is the CEO of Jay Robb Enterprises—a multi-million dollar corporation (founded in 1988) that is famous for its high-quality, outrageously delicious protein powder formulas. Jay Robb products and books are sold in thousands of health food stores and gyms across the nation.

Jay is the author of the top-selling book *The Fat Burning Diet*, a feature columnist for *Natural Bodybuilding* magazine, and a contributing writer for *Men's Exercise*, *Women's Exercise*, and *Exercise for Men Only*.

The Jay Robb Corporation also produces the Jay Robb *Health-E-Newsletter,* which is featured on the company website: www.JayRobb.com.

Jay Robb has devoted his life to God. He is happily married, has one son, and lives in La Costa, California—on San Diego's beautiful North County coastline.

"Be still, and know that I am God."
—Psalm 46:10

Chapter 1
The Secret to Burning Fat

"'God, help me!' I cried out in desperation. I had no idea that the answer to my prayer would profoundly change my life and, quite possibly, the life of millions."

My fat burning journey began one day in 1978, following a routine trip to the gym. I was performing the inclined bench press, and on repetition number three, I lost my strength and the bar came crashing down on my chest. Bam! Two guys had to pull the bar off my chest to keep it from crushing me. At the point I was freed of the bar, I noticed how weak and shaky I had become. The room was spinning, and I felt dizzy and disoriented. It was frightening because I didn't know what was wrong with me. I had never in my life felt this way. In a panic, I managed to find my gym bag and headed straight for the door.

I honestly don't recall driving home that day, but I made it there and inserted the key in the door with my weak, shaky right hand. I opened the door, entered, and slammed it shut quickly. Feeling safe at home, I advanced three steps forward into my living room—when suddenly my knees buckled. I collapsed on the floor, landing flat on my back. In total fear, I lay helpless, looking up at the ceiling, which appeared to be spinning out of control. Petrified—the tears streamed down both sides of my face and pooled onto the hardwood floor beneath my head. My body was drained of all energy. It was as if I was nailed to the floor. Suddenly, the thought entered my mind that I was experiencing a nervous breakdown. I was devastated. A crossroads moment, you might say.

The Fat Burning Diet

I was raised in a Christian household where we learned at a very young age to pray when the burden of life was too much to bear. Could there be a more perfect moment? There I was—completely helpless—and paralyzed from fear. I mustered up enough strength to position my palms together and prayed. This was not one of those "bless me and my life" perfunctory prayers; this prayer came from my heart. "God, help me!" I cried out in desperation. I had no idea that the answer to my prayer would profoundly change my life and, quite possibly, the life of millions.

"God, help me, please. Allow my energy, health, and strength to return," I pleaded. "If you reveal the secret to regaining my health and well-being, I promise to share this information with the world. I will make it my life's mission, and I will give you *all* the glory."

Suddenly, the room stopped spinning, and I was able to sit up. At that moment, I looked up toward the heavens and felt an assuredness that my prayer *was* heard from above. From that moment on, I was a changed person—a man on a mission!

> "I would have despaired and perished unless Your laws had been my deepest delight. I will never lay aside Your laws, for You have used them to restore my joy and health. I am Yours!"
> —Psalm 119:92-94

The Lord *did* restore my health, completely. And I was led to a deeper understanding of God's dietary laws that allowed me to find my way back to health—*but it didn't happen overnight.* And, frankly, I'm glad it didn't. The journey deepened my appreciation for God's blessing more than ever.

This journey to discovering the root cause of my health problem took over 10 years. Shortly after my collapse, I was diagnosed with *reactive hypoglycemia*, the medical term for "low blood sugar." Mood swings, anger, depression, energy slumps, exhaustion, and chronic fatigue can all be traced to this simple blood sugar disorder. I wanted to treat the symptoms, but I was even more interested in learning how to prevent my body from developing future complications.

While *my* reaction was severe, not typical, millions of Americans every day experience symptoms from mild hypoglycemia (mood swings, mild depression, anxiety, and fatigue). *Hypoglycemia* is a condition indicating "very low (below normal) sugar in the bloodstream." Without an adequate blood sugar supply, the body can weaken and the brain can become confused. Hypoglycemia can be *chronic* (constant) or *reactive* (sporadic).

"Left untreated, hypoglycemia may become diabetes in a matter of years" were the words that came straight out of my doctor's mouth after he confirmed my condition. His diagnosis came after I completed an extensive six-hour glucose tolerance test in his office (refer to blood sugar charts on pages 60-63). He was helpful to a point—yet I firmly believed God would provide me with the treatment I needed to overcome this disease and regain my health and strength. And God delivered!

At the time of *this* writing, I am now 50 years old and healthier and happier than ever. For over two decades, God has blessed me with wisdom and revealed His dietary laws and truths that I believe are the answer to optimum health. If a man's success is defined by finding his purpose in life and fulfilling that purpose—then I am a very wealthy man. It is truly a labor of love helping others find the health and peace of mind they have always dreamt about.

So what *does* hypoglycemia have to do with burning fat? *Everything!* In my quest to eliminate hypoglycemia, I made three discoveries about burning fat.

DISCOVERY #1:
By allowing the body to burn fat frequently, you naturally avoid

any possibility of developing diabetes Type 2 or hypoglycemia (low blood sugar).

DISCOVERY #2:
The body's fuel of choice is FAT, not carbohydrate—a concept totally different from what I was taught in school.

DISCOVERY #3:
On The Fat Burning Diet, you can safely eat the carbs you love and still burn fat up to 24 hours a day—with or without exercise.

In these pages, I will reveal the ultimate diet for burning fat. I will also explain why low-carb diets and high-carb diets can be ineffective for permanent weight management. But when you OFFSET high-carb meals with low-carb meals, you get what I call "The Fat Burning Diet"—a diet you can follow for a lifetime!

"Success follows what you do. There is no other way to be successful."
—Malcolm Forbes

Chapter 2
The 3 Most Popular Diets and Why They ONLY Work Short-term

"My name is Sherlock Holmes. It
is my business to know what
other people don't know."
—Sir Arthur Conan Doyle

Do you feel like a snapdragon? No snap and everything draggin'! Have you tried every diet on the planet, but all you ever lost was your patience? If you answered "yes" to either of those questions, then The Fat Burning Diet is for you.

Two haircutting salons were in serious competition with each other. One salon put up a sign advertising haircuts for $2. The other salon across the street, not to be outdone, posted a sign that stated: "We Repair $2 Haircuts!"

My job with this book is to repair $2 diets. A low-fat high-carbo-hydrate diet is what I call a "$2 diet." An extreme low-carb diet is also what I call a "$2 diet." Why are they $2 diets? Because they both offer a quick fix and are not designed to deliver results for a lifetime. Not to worry, however. I am here to repair them both. Let me explain.

"The *real* difference
between men is energy."
—Fuller

DIET #1: The Low-Carb Diet (Ketosis-inducing)

In the early '70s, an American doctor made famous a low-carb eating plan that could force the body to burn fat by radically limiting all forms of carbohydrate. Once all carbohydrate reserves were depleted in the body, the body was then able to switch from a glucose burning state to a fat burning state (medically termed *ketosis*) 100 percent of the time. This was not a new diet, yet this doctor became world renowned for refining and promoting it. The diet worked wonders for rapid weight loss with participants dropping weight almost overnight and often without hunger. This low-carb diet may sound miraculous and just what you are looking for, but I am here to tell you this style of eating has some serious flaws. Let me explain further.

Low-Carb Replay

In the early '90s, this same extreme low-carb diet re-emerged after lying dormant since the mid-to-late '70s. Once again, dieters were encouraged to severely cut carbs and load up on fat and protein. They could wallow in butter, cream cheese, macadamia nuts, whole eggs, and juicy steaks while melting away fat without effort. In general, and in my opinion, cutting one's carbohydrate intake is healthy and effective as a means of losing weight—for short periods of time—but not for a lifetime. Severely cutting carbs is magical for a few days—but not for weeks, months, or years.

Below are Some Potential Drawbacks to an Extreme Low-Carb Ketosis-inducing Diet:

1. It can become extremely monotonous and boring due to the limited variety of foods to choose from.

2. Binging can take place as a rebound effect of restricting carbohydrate for too long.

3. It can slow one's metabolism because of *chronic glycogen*

24

debt (severely diminished levels of stored muscle starch). When the body is short on reserves, it can trigger a metabolic slowdown because the body thinks it is starving.

4. It can lead to constipation and a low level of *lactobacteria* (the friendly bacteria) in the colon. An extreme low-carb diet is usually low in natural fiber and lactobacteria food because it is almost void of *lactose* (milk sugar) and starches and low in fresh fruits and vegetables.

5. A ketogenic diet does not allow its participants to rise to their peak shape if they are exercising regularly or if they are athletic. The muscles require carbohydrate for running, fast jogging, sprinting, weight training, cycling, swimming, or any activity that requires quick movements.

6. It can also be too low in antioxidants, Vitamin C, and the cancer prevention nutrients found in fresh fruits and vegetables.

7. A high-fat high-protein diet can be extremely high in calories. Fat contains nine calories per gram, so a pint of cream or stick of butter can radically add to your daily calorie intake. Calories DO count. Many extreme low-carb dieters have become discouraged when their weight loss came to a screeching halt after a month or two. One explanation for the extreme low-carb diet no longer working is because the calorie intake no longer allowed for weight loss—no matter how low the carb intake was. High-calorie diets can make you fat—period! And a low-carb ketogenic diet is no exception.

In my opinion, cutting carbs is a good thing, but cutting them for too long is not. **For burning fat, cutting carbs is critical, but you must know when to avoid carbs and when to eat them.** That is what The Fat Burning Diet is all about.

DIET #2: The High-Carb Diet (Low in fat)

On the other end of the spectrum is the low-fat high-carbohy-drate diet that was extremely popular throughout the '80s and early '90s. The secret to that diet was to trim away almost all fat from your diet and eat 70% or more of your calories in the form of complex carbohydrates.

As fat intake is lowered radically, so are the calories. **Lowering calories can induce weight loss but not specifically fat loss.** Your body cannot readily burn fat in the presence of *insulin* (the hormone secreted by your pancreas that has several func-tions—with its primary purpose being the regulation of blood sugar levels). Insulin is secreted whenever your blood sugar lev-els rise above a certain point. Once insulin is secreted, all fat burning stops, and your body switches from a fat burning state to a *sugar* (glucose) burning state.

A low-fat high-carbohydrate diet can cause your body to produce high concentrations of insulin necessary to control the continu-al rise in blood sugar levels due to the amount of carbohydrate being ingested. Once insulin is secreted, all fat burning stops, and your body begins burning sugar—from various sources in the body—instead of drawing energy from your fat cells. Your body will continue to burn sugar, not fat, as long as sugar lev-els are high in the bloodstream and insulin is present.

A woman with a very short haircut made the low-fat high-carb diet popular in the early '90s, and millions jumped on the band-wagon, just as they did with the low-carb ketogenic diet craze.

At first, the low-fat high-carb diet works like a miracle. But over time, many low-fat high-carb dieters fail to lose weight and actu-ally start gaining weight! Why? I believe it is from the over-con-sumption of carbohydrate in the form of grains, starches, sug-ars, fruit, and carbs. Combine this with the action of *insulin* (which is your fat storing hormone), and you get weight gain, not weight loss.

For low-fat high-carbohydrate dieters, there can only be one way to make that diet work. EXERCISE! This dieter must always be in motion to burn up the sugar in his or her bloodstream. Should this dieter ever rest, take a day off, or fail to exercise, he or she could rapidly pack on extra weight and perhaps experience some nasty bouts with hypoglycemia. The weight gain and blood sugar challenges would be caused by the continual rise in blood sugar levels from continual high-carb eating.

Additionally, eating carbohydrates without fat allows the carbohydrate to convert to blood sugar quicker than if fats are eaten at the same time. Thus the low-fat high-carb dieter could be constantly getting a sugar rush from the high-carbohydrate content of the foods being consumed. Over time, this could lead to hypoglycemia and *adrenal fatigue* (primarily caused by the overproduction of adrenalin to repeatedly raise low blood sugar conditions). The problem lies not with the high-carb diet itself. The problem arises as the duration of the diet increases—which is the same problem the low-carb ketogenic dieter faces.

DIET #3: The Modified High-Carb Diet
(Balancing carbohydrate, protein, and fat to burn fat)

Around 1995, four years after The Fat Burning Diet was first released, a new diet emerged that purported to have the answer to permanent weight loss. This diet cited specific ratios of carbohydrate to protein to fat, with the carbohydrate portion being 40%, making it a modified high-carb diet. The fat portion of the diet was set at 30%, which was something new to America—adding a twist to high-carb eating. The plan also emphasized the importance of eating enough protein each day. But this diet was flawed.

First, because the dieter was instructed to eat exact protein, fat, and carbohydrate percentages at each meal, it was very challenging to consume a perfectly balanced meal. Second, on this rigid diet, 40% of the calories came from carbohydrate—

which was great for athletes and active individuals but terrible for office workers and moderately active folks (who represent a significant percentage of America's population).

Third, this diet included wheat and grains that a significant portion of the population may be allergic to. Consequently, this new carbohydrate-, protein-, and fat-balancing diet could only work for those who were: a) very active (exercising an hour or more daily), b) willing to calculate the exact percentages of protein, fat, and carbs at each meal, and c) not allergic or sensitive to grains, wheat, or gluten. All in all, this new diet was still a high-carb diet; yet, as you will see, eating high-carb meals ALL the time is not the answer.

Below are Some Challenges the High-Carb Dieter May Face:

1. Fatigue can occur just by consuming excess carbohydrate, especially the *wrong types of carbohydrate*—refined wheat, pasta, white bread, processed breakfast cereals, and the majority of grains are considered "bad" or "avoidable" carbohydrates. Eating high levels of refined carbohydrate stimulates the release of insulin, which allows tryptophan to reach the brain in high concentrations. Tryptophan in the brain can readily convert to the brain chemical neurotransmitter *serotonin*, which can be very sedating. In fact, many low-fat high-carb dieters who consume processed grains—pasta is one of the greatest offenders—as their primary carbohydrate source find themselves yawning frequently and feeling tired much of the time.

2. Weight gain is common unless the high-carb eater is an endurance athlete. Endurance athletes exercising 2-4 hours a day can usually burn up the excess glucose created from the high-carb intake. But for those who exercise moderately (30 minutes a day or less), a high-carb diet can spell d-i-s-a-s-t-er and promote a thick middle.

3. Muscle tissue can be sacrificed on a low-fat high-carb diet if

the protein intake is too low. Adding protein to an extreme low-fat high-carb diet can also spell w-e-i-g-h-t g-a-i-n due to the extra calories and digestive slowdown caused by consuming too much protein with starches. In my experience and professional opinion, protein intake needs to be approximately 15-20% of the total calories of a high-carb meal to achieve maximum digestive power.

4. Carbohydrate addiction can occur because 40-70% or more of calories are coming from carbs at nearly EVERY MEAL.

5. Wheat and other gluten-containing grains are often consumed regularly, and this can lead to food allergies and weight gain. Millions of Americans may be allergic to wheat and/or gluten in the wheat. (Wheat, oats, rye, and barley contain the protein *gluten* which many individuals cannot break down properly. Undigested gluten can irritate and damage the delicate intestinal lining in those who are gluten intolerant.) Pasta is one of the favorite foods of the high-carb dieter. In my opinion, it is also one of the most allergenic and fattening foods on this planet.

6. Grains become a staple food for most high-carb dieters. Grains are what farmers feed their cattle to fatten them for market. Hmmm. Think about it. Grains require a lot of insulin to manage, which explains why cows (and humans) can become fat. Moooooooo! Head 'em up; move 'em out!

7. Low-fat diets can be low in the essential fatty acids (Omega-3 and Omega-6) category. Fats are essential. If you don't get them in your diet, you can develop a serious nutritional deficiency that can make you sick. Should this deficiency go on for too long, death can occur.

Perhaps you can relate to some of these findings. Americans typically hop from one diet to the next because they don't experience success for one reason or another. The above-referenced list offers an explanation as to why individuals are still in search of the perfect diet. Both camps—low-carb dieters and high-carb dieters—have argued their viewpoint and praised the benefits of each style of eating. But one thing was missing in their discussion:

What would happen if you combined the low-carb diet with the high-carb diet? In other words, could you have the best of both worlds and get the benefit of both diets?

Yes, you can! Now let me show you how easy it is to follow this time-proven revolutionary way of eating. You're going to love it!

"Greater is he who conquers himself than he who conquers a thousand."
—Buddha

Chapter 3
The Fat Burning Diet

Glycogen Management
is the Key to Success

A low-carb diet works fabulous for a day or two until the body runs out of stored glycogen. Then it can begin to sputter as it switches to burning ketones. Similarly, the high-carb diet works great for a day or two until glycogen levels are filled to capacity—at which time all excess *glucose* (blood sugar) can be converted to fat.

The Real Secret to Permanent Weight Management

Burning fat consistently, while maintaining high energy and physical power, requires one day of low-carb eating followed by one day of high-carb eating. Then simply repeat the cycle each week, with Sunday allowing for both types of eating.

NOTE: You will consume three meals a day: breakfast, lunch, and dinner. In order for The Fat Burning Diet to lend spectacular results, you will refrain from eating ALL snacks—until your weight is at a normal level or unless you are extremely active. Because of the great addiction we, as a nation, have to carbohydrates, this step may seem unattainable. A TIP: Liken this carbohydrate addiction to cigarette smoking. Once the *habit* is broken, the *desire* for foods that often make you feel hyper, puffy, stuffed, gassy or cause acne or weight gain will go away. It's really that simple. You have control over what goes in your mouth each and every time you open it.

The Fat Burning Diet

The Fat Burning Diet Meal Patterns:

Monday: Low-carb breakfast, lunch & dinner.
Tuesday: High-carb breakfast, lunch & dinner.
Wednesday: Low-carb breakfast, lunch & dinner.
Thursday: High-carb breakfast, lunch & dinner.
Friday: Low-carb breakfast, lunch & dinner.
Saturday: High-carb breakfast, lunch & FREE MEAL dinner.
Sunday: Low-carb breakfast and lunch / high-carb dinner.
                        Repeat this eating pattern.

Why does this style of eating work so well? There are many, many reasons, but "glycogen" is the real secret.

GLP (Glycogen Loading Principle)

Glycogen is "stored muscle starch." Your body will convert and store excess blood glucose as glycogen as long as there is room to store it. If glycogen levels are full, your body will simply convert excess glucose into body fat. This is the main reason a high-carb diet doesn't work over a long period of time.

The secret to eating carbs safely, without them converting to fat, is to make sure glycogen levels are *never* full. How do you do that? It's easy. You cut carbs. Cutting carbs is the easiest way to burn down your glycogen levels. Exercise can help but should not be relied upon for glycogen management. Your diet is the best way to manage glycogen levels.

The average active person can store approximately 400 grams of carbohydrate in the form of muscle and liver glycogen. 400 grams! This is a fact that the low-carb ketogenic diet supporter does not want you to know. Four hundred grams of carbohydrate is the equivalent of approximately 16 bowls of oatmeal, 50 rice cakes, 40 pancakes, 36 slices of wheat bread, 40 cups of steamed green beans, 10 cups of cooked corn, 50 cups of steamed zucchini, or 19 medium-size apples.

Let me make this point about glycogen crystal clear. If you have room to store glycogen, then excess carbohydrate is usually converted to glycogen instead of *triglyceride* (fat that is destined to be stored in your fat cells).

> The secret to weight management and fat burning is to simply *monitor your glycogen levels* through carbohydrate control.

Exercise helps in the management of glycogen, but your diet is the most effective means of depleting and loading glycogen. And with approximately 400 grams of carbohydrate to play with, you have plenty of room for error in this equation. This is the last thing the extreme low-carb diet advocate wants you to hear.

The last thing the high-carbohydrate supporter wants you to know is that once you have filled your glycogen levels to the top, then ALL excess carbohydrate consumed from that point on can be converted to fat. Soon all that extra fat (*triglyceride*) may be filling the fat cells throughout your body.

Stop the Fighting!

The Fat Burning Diet ends all fighting between the diet experts. The Fat Burning Diet makes everyone right. Low-carb diets DO work—but only for short periods of time until glycogen levels are depleted. High-carb diets DO work—but only for short periods of time until glycogen levels are full. The secret is to simply mesh the two styles of eating together (in a very unique way) so that you get the best of both worlds—a diet you can live with for the rest of your life.

Now that you know the secret to staying lean for life, let me share with you the basic overview of The Fat Burning Diet. I have also included one full week of sample menus so you can start burning fat immediately.

Glycogen Depleting/Loading Chart
for Traditional Fat Burning Diet

 Indicates available liver and muscle glycogen.
(Note: Actual glycogen depletion and loading varies with each individual and is dependent on many factors—including exercise and the amount of calories and carbohydrate consumed.)

One Low-Carb Day

Beginning of Day 1	Noon of Day 1	5pm of Day 1	10pm of Day 1
	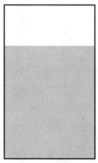	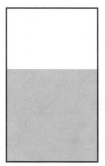	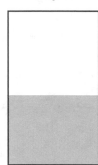
Glycogen almost full	Glycogen depletes	Glycogen depletes	Glycogen is low

One High-Carb Day

Beginning of Day 2	Noon of Day 2	5pm of Day 2	10pm of Day 2
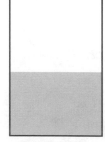			
Glycogen is low	Glycogen refills	Glycogen refills	Glycogen almost full

Glycogen Depleting/Loading Chart
for Bodybuilders

 Indicates available liver and muscle glycogen.
(Note: Actual glycogen depletion and loading varies with each individual and is dependent on many factors—including exercise and the amount of calories and carbohydrate consumed.)

Two Low-Carb Days

Beginning of Day 1	10pm of Day 1	Noon of Day 2	10pm of Day 2

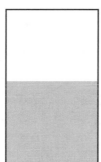 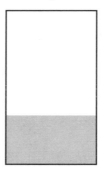 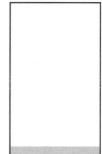

Glycogen almost full	Glycogen depletes	Glycogen depletes	Glycogen very low

One Very High-Carb Day

Beginning of Day 3	Noon of Day 3	5pm of Day 3	10pm of Day 3

   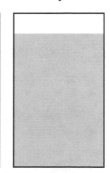

Glycogen very low	Glycogen refills	Glycogen refills	Glycogen almost full

The Fat Burning Diet

OVERVIEW OF THE DIET

The Fat Burning Diet is Unique and Effective Because You:

1. —utilize Jay Robb's unique food-combining principles—eating high-carb meals separate from low-carb meals—thus ensuring the best digestion possible.

2. —deplete glycogen levels on low-carb days. Then after a day or so, you begin eating higher-carb meals to replenish it. Then you glycogen deplete again with low-carb meals, and repeat the cycle.

3. —get to consume high-fat protein meals on some days and high-carb low-fat meals on other days. In other words, you get to indulge in the best of BOTH worlds.

4. —get to eat anything you desire for one hour a week (Jay's FREE MEAL). I suggest Saturday evening.

5. —never feel deprived. On The Fat Burning Diet, the menu encompasses a wide variety of foods, including some carbohydrate-rich foods and fatty foods.

6. —can ensure you are eating enough alkaline fruits and vegetables by checking your urine with pH test strips and then altering the amount of alkaline foods you will eat based on the test and your unique needs.

7. —can lose excess fat even if you are NOT exercising. Yes, that's right. You can burn fat without lifting a finger. You WILL be encouraged to lift a fork to your lips, however.

8. —will feel satisfied, not only because of improved digestion, but because you will be functioning daily in a state of fat burning. You will also produce well-formed, almost odorless, bowel movements.

9. —can kiss gas, bloating, indigestion, constipation, diarrhea, and other digestive disorders goodbye forever!

10. —may no longer need to wear deodorant because of improved digestion and the cleansing effect of fruits and vegetables.

Guidelines for Following The Fat Burning Diet:

1. ALL meals should be either a low-carb meal or a high-carb meal.

2. You will consume one day of low-carb meals followed by one day of high-carb meals, and then repeat the cycle. It's that easy.

3. Eat only THREE meals a day. After years of testing, I conclude that snacks *can* interfere with digestion and add extra calories that are not needed. Instead, eat three solid meals that are adequate in calories to hold you for approximately 5-6 hours. A simple schedule is to eat breakfast between 6am and 8am, lunch between 11am and 1pm, and dinner between 6pm and 8pm. NO SNACKING or late night eating is allowed. (Trust me on this.) You will be very satisfied with my program and the foods you are eating. The three-meals-a-day plan also saves you time and money because you no longer have to shop, pay for, and prepare snacks. NOTE: If you are an athlete, physical laborer, or endurance athlete, you may be able to include snacks in your diet once your body fat returns to a normal level.

4. Starches—in the form of potatoes, yams, squash, brown rice, and sweet potatoes—are consumed on high-carb days only. NO starches are consumed on low-carb days. Naturally occurring carbs from vegetables, yogurt, sweet dairy whey, and small amounts of fresh fruit are the only carbohydrates consumed on low-carb days.

5. Your fat intake will naturally be higher on low-carb days and

lower on high-carb days.

6. On low-carb days, you will consume approximately 30-45% protein, 30-45% healthy fats, and 10-25% carbohydrate.

7. On high-carb days, you will consume approximately 15-25% protein, 15-30% healthy fats, and 45-70% carbohydrate.

8. Eat one <u>extra large</u> RAW salad every day. This salad should contain approximately 3-5 cups of mixed raw low-carb vegetables. On low-carb days, this salad may contain avocado, cheese, nuts, eggs, egg whites, your choice of meat, and/or 1-3 tablespoons of raw apple cider vinegar or your dressing of choice. On high-carb days, this salad may contain carrots, corn, peas, avocado, raw nuts, and up to 2 ounces of meat, cheese, or 2 hard-boiled eggs. When people see me sit down to consume my daily salad, they often comment that it looks like a salad prepared for three to four people. In my opinion, you can never eat too many raw vegetables.

9. Protein and vegetables are the main calories to focus on during low-carb days. On high-carb days, protein should be limited to approximately 2-3 ounces of meat or 2-3 eggs at each meal so that starch digestion is not inhibited.

10. It is easy to be a *vegetarian* (lacto-ovo) on The Fat Burning Diet. You can make the diet vegetarian by eating other protein sources—such as eggs, dairy, whey protein powder, egg white protein powder, and soy protein powder—rather than meat.

11. The more active you are, the more carbohydrate you will need and can consume safely without storing fat.

12. If you become hungry between meals, drink 12-16 ounces of water. Hunger can actually be your body's way of telling you it is thirsty. Drink water and watch your hunger dissipate. You may also add a squeeze of lime or lemon and a dash of granulated stevia powder to your water to create a refreshing taste.

Although I am not in favor of snacking unless you are a very active person, if you feel you are extremely hungry between meals, even though you are drinking water, you may try munching on baby carrots or raw vegetables as a mid-morning or mid-afternoon snack.

13. Do not skip meals. Skipping meals can seriously slow your metabolism. Your body demands food on a regular basis, so eat your three main meals every day. **Skipping meals too frequently can actually cause you to gain weight.**

14. Fats must be consumed for good health because they are essential; limit them because they are also high in calories.

15. Start every day with Jay's Lemonade or Jay's Vitamin C Tea. These alkaline drinks may also be consumed with meals. Jay's Lemonade is made with 12 ounces of water and the fresh juice of ½ lime or lemon. Jay's Vitamin C Tea is made with 12 ounces of water and 1½ teaspoons of acerola berry powder (a rich source of Vitamin C). Add ½ teaspoon granulated stevia powder to create a sweet-tasting drink. (Stevia is not classed as a "sweetener" but creates a sweet taste when mixed with tart foods and acid fruits.)

16. Drink at least a half gallon of pure water daily.

17. During the warmer months of the year, when melons are ripe and prolific, you may consume them as the first meal of the day on high-carb days if your body fat levels are at or near the range you prefer. Do not mix any other fruit or food with melons. Eat them alone and as the first food of the day only.

18. To avoid constipation, gas, bloating, and to help feed the friendly bacteria in your colon, consume for breakfast—three or more mornings a week—16 ounces of nonfat or low-fat plain yogurt mixed with 2 tablespoons of sweet dairy whey and 2 tablespoons of ground flax seeds (golden flax seeds are the best). You may also have one piece (or serving) of fresh fruit

with this mixture—consuming low-carb fruit on low-carb days and high-carb fruit on high-carb days. I always mix a little granulated stevia powder with the yogurt and sweet dairy whey to make it taste sweet like pudding. I also consume 1-2 capsules of a lactase enzyme to assist in digesting the lactose in the whey. (Sweet dairy whey can also be mixed into your favorite protein drink.)

19. When dining at restaurants, simply select low-carb foods or high-carb foods on the menu, and enjoy!

20. Take your temperature orally 2-3 times daily between meals to ensure your metabolism is up to speed. Your temperature, between the hours of 9am and 7pm, should be approximately 98.6 degrees Fahrenheit. A reading of 97.9 or less could indicate a slow metabolism. (See Chapter 16 for more details.)

21. Salt and salty foods should be avoided. Instead, choose fresh foods, low-salt foods, and use a potassium-based salt substitute to season your foods. Salt (*sodium chloride*), in the form of table salt, can cause bloating and weight gain. *Natural sodium that occurs in whole foods—such as egg whites, sea vegetables, and fish—is an essential mineral and different from sodium chloride (table salt), which is a refined product.*

22. Condiments are allowed in moderation, but try to always select low-salt low-carb sugar-free brands.

23. Caffeine, alcohol, and all non-prescription drugs should be limited—especially avoid over-the-counter diet supplements that contain herbal stimulants. Caffeine-free tea, herbal teas, and coffee are okay. Alcohol, in limited amounts, is best consumed at high-carb meals or during your once-a-week free meal. I often consume a small glass of wine in the evening during a high-carb meal. Moderation is the key.

What to Expect from Following The Fat Burning Diet:

1. Your body fat should plunge to a normally low level and stay there for the rest of your life. The magic comes from eating low-carb foods and high-carb foods at separate meals or on separate days.

2. Your energy levels should be at an all-time high—i.e., no more mid-morning fatigue or afternoon brain fog.

3. Fatigue, anxiety, depression, moods swings, and bad moods should become a thing of the past.

4. If you are a diabetic, blood sugar levels should be easier than ever to monitor and control.

5. Your bowel movements should become effortless, odorless, and not require the traditional cleanup with toilet paper. In other words, your feces will leave your body easily, without offensive odors and a messy texture. This will be due to the use of sweet dairy whey, which proliferates lactobacteria, and the eating of high-carb foods and low-carb foods at separate meals or on separate days.

6. You should be able to eliminate the need for deodorant once your body can clean house on The Fat Burning Diet. In my experience, a toxic colon, poor food combinations, and too much saturated fat (excess fat consumption is known to cause underarm odor) can lead to underarm odor. Since 1978, after cleansing and feeding the lactobacteria in my colon and consuming only natural foods, I have not had a need for deodorant. Any time my diet contains a limited amount of fruits and vegetables and too much fat, or unwholesome foods, the underarm odor will return to remind me to consume only natural foods. It may take you several months to clean house so you can toss away your deodorant—but it *can* happen once your body is a clean machine!

7. Your urine should become relatively clear and odorless. This will be due to the high consumption of pure water, efficient digestion, timely elimination, a high lactobacteria count in your colon, and the consumption of fruits and vegetables in ample quantities. NOTE: If you are consuming a vitamin supplement that contains Vitamin B_2, your urine may turn bright yellow when any excess of this vitamin is excreted.

8. Your urine should test alkaline at a pH range between 7.0 and 7.4 at least 50% of the time (test daily with pH test strips). Always test immediately upon awakening or between meals. This test indicates if you are eating enough alkaline-based foods—especially fruits and vegetables.

9. If your urine tests acidic more than 50% of the time, then you need to focus on eating as much of the alkaline foods as possible (alkaline foods on the food list are clearly marked—see pages 53-58). This translates to eating loads of vegetables, including extra large salads made with a variety of low-carb vegetables. On high-carb days, break out the juicer and make as much fresh vegetable juice as you desire. Continue focusing on alkaline foods until your urine tests alkaline at least 50% of the time. Taking coral minerals (coral calcium, coral magnesium, and trace minerals) can also help provide your body with more alkaline minerals to add to its reserves.

10. If you are diabetic, have chronic fatigue, or are experiencing hypoglycemia or reactive hypoglycemia, then you should monitor your glucose levels daily with a glucose monitor. (Always check with your doctor first concerning all health issues. See Chapter 12 for more information on diabetes.)

11. If you are an insulin-dependent diabetic, you may require very little insulin, or perhaps none at all, on low-carb days. Taking insulin on low-carb days could lower your glucose levels significantly, so be aware of this. Utilizing The Fat Burning Diet principles can cut your insulin needs in half because of carbohydrate restriction and alkaline eating patterns. (Always check

with your doctor first concerning all health issues, including your diet.)

Five Additional Tips to Ensure Success:

1. Monitor your fat-loss progress by testing your body fat levels with a good pair of home-use digital calipers, or have your body fat tested professionally at your local doctor's office or fitness center. DO NOT measure your progress with a doctor's scale or bathroom scale. My desire is to teach you how to lose excess fat—not muscle, water, or bone. Weight loss could be anything. Fat loss is *fat loss* and is easily determined by body fat testing.

2. Breathe! That's right. Become aware of your breathing, and inhale deeper and more frequently. Tension and stress have a tendency to make us hold our breath, which can starve our cells of vital oxygen. **Fat cannot be used as fuel unless oxygen is present; consistent deep breathing is critical to burning fat and being healthy.** Being aerobically fit also assists fat burning because oxygen is more abundant and is utilized more readily due to conditioning and training.

3. Exercise at least three days a week doing something you enjoy. If you don't belong to a fitness club, then join one today. If you are not fond of gyms, then go outside and run or power walk. Buy a set of weights and a small bench, and train at home. Or go surfing, cycling, hiking, or mountain climbing. Enroll in an aerobics class. The secret is to elevate your heart rate to 70-85% of its maximum level for at least 20 minutes, three times a week. You must also lift weights (training all the major muscles) at least one day a week to strengthen the muscles and ensure bone density is maximized.

4. Before you start The Fat Burning Diet, check with your doctor, and get a complete physical, including blood work. This will be your starting point. Note your triglyceride level, cholesterol level, body weight, temperature, and body fat level. Then have new blood work performed every three months, and note all

changes and improvements.

5. CALORIES COUNT! No matter how perfect you are eating, if you are consuming too many calories, you will not *lose weight*. You may even gain weight. **On the other hand, if you eat too few calories, your body may fear it is starving and automatically slow your metabolism so that you don't lose any weight.** I have had several clients who cut their calories so low they actually started gaining weight because their metabolism shut down.

"If you are asleep at the wheel,
wake up and let God drive."
—The Author

Chapter 4
The Most Important Chapter in this Book

The Secret to Successful Dieting

As a nutrition counselor, over the past 25 years I have looked into the eyes of thousands of dieters. Many of the eyes I looked into reflected excitement and enthusiasm while others projected sadness, depictive of the hopelessness they felt. Many were hungry for success, but still many lacked the internal motivation to succeed with the new diet I would eventually share with them.

There is one thing I have learned about dieting success. An individual must be genuinely and seriously motivated, or there will be no lasting results. If there is not a burning passion to succeed in the heart of a dieter, then he or she will simply start the new diet only to abandon it within 30 days (and sometimes at the first sign of weakness or temptation).

You may now be asking, "How do *I* get motivated about losing weight so that I am able to follow The Fat Burning Diet for the rest of my life?" The answer to this is twofold. First, you must discover your TRUE purpose for getting in shape. And, second, you must ask for help each day. Sure, this sounds simple, but allow me to explain further so that you completely understand what you need to do to achieve the success you have always dreamed of.

There is no question as to the effectiveness of The Fat Burning Diet. Since 1991 it has helped thousands upon thousands of individuals lose weight and keep it off. Those individuals who found success with my diet all shared one thing in common—a strong desire to succeed. In other words, they had a purpose for losing weight and keeping it off. Thousands of *other* individuals have also been introduced to my diet. Many of them found initial success with the program, but, because of a lack of motivation, they soon reverted back to their old eating habits even though they knew the diet worked and improved their health. To put it bluntly, you must have a serious reason for getting in shape, or all your efforts will be in vain. Vanity is where the *real* problem begins.

If you desire to lose weight for self-centered reasons, then chances are you will not stick with the program because it will require you to develop and maintain a hefty ego. "What's in it for ME?" is one of the most self-destructive questions you can ask yourself in life. Anything done for YOURSELF often excludes others and puts YOU in the spotlight. Getting in shape for summer, losing weight for a reunion or cruise, or shedding those extra pounds to attract a mate, can all be shallow, self-centered goals that can produce short-term results. But when you are getting in shape for reasons other than your own personal gain, the real magic begins. Let me explain.

> "We should be as attractive as we possibly can be for God; He gets all the glory when we do."

Imagine, for a moment, that our existence here on earth is a game. What is the purpose of this game? Let's imagine it is to *find happiness.* The question is: Are you truly happy? If you were to ask this question to 100 individuals, you might get varied answers, and most might respond superficially, "Yes, I'm basically happy." But if you were to look deep into the eyes of these people, you might see the contrary. If you could see into their hearts, you might see that they are actually very sad, angry, hurt, or lost.

In reality, life IS about finding happiness, and true happiness is the key to success at dieting or anything else you do in life. But how *do* we find true happiness? You don't. Happiness is not something you must find. It is something you must realize. Happiness is never *lost*, so there is no need to search for it. Happiness is experienced when you are connected with the Creator. Without this connection, life has little or no meaning and often becomes purposeless.

> "We all want to be famous people, and the moment we want to *be* something, we are no longer free."
> —Krishnamurti

Everything you do for "you" can be a shallow experience that can lead to addictions, sadness, frustration, and pain. Why? It's simple. Life is not complete when you fill your days thinking about yourself—instead of God. "You" are high maintenance whether you admit it or not. Just look around you, and admire all the "stuff" in your life. Stuff? Yes, stuff. Cars, an entertainment center, tape players, CDs, CD players, DVD players, clothes, jewelry, watches, golf clubs, paintings, balls, bats, surfboards, computers, books, magazines, computer games, the internet, magazines, cell phones, adding machines, tools, cosmetics, perfume, nail polish, furniture, gizmos, and gadgets! If you haven't acquired all these things yet, chances are you have a desire for or may think you need them. The question is: What is the purpose for having all these "things" in your life?

Let me be clear on this point. *There is nothing wrong with having "things."* It's the purpose for having your "things" that you may want to examine. For many, toys become the perfect pacifier or panacea. It can be the distraction that keeps you from actually engaging in life and experiencing some of the basic joys it offers. The harsh reality is that human beings have a tendency to become self-centered materialists.

Right now you may be taken aback, or even insulted, as you read this chapter, but please hear me out. That is not my intent.

I am trying to illustrate a very salient point as we strive to understand why it is so hard for us to stick with a diet program on a long-term basis. What I have to say has every potentiality to change your life and inspire you to find happiness and dietary success once and for all.

"It takes one to know one..."

During the 1970s, I was self-consumed. My life was all about ME. From the outside looking in, however, most would think of me as having it all together. I was living with an attractive woman. I had a fantastic muscular body. I was debt-free and in the prime of my life, yet I was not happy—though I tried to convince myself that I was. *My day was all about Jay.* I was self-consumed with pleasure, living in sin, and, as a result, my life turned into a living hell.

Despite my external appearance, I was miserable inside because I thought I could *find* happiness if I had a beautiful woman, big muscles, and the freedom to indulge in pleasure. I took care of "yours truly" every opportunity that arose. Ironically, the more I focused on Jay, the more depressed I felt—which drove me to a pattern of drinking more, eating more, chasing women, and engaging in self-destructive habits.

Then one day in 1978, my life collapsed when I collapsed. My body and mind could no longer take the abuse I was inflicting upon it, and I went down for the count. Out of sheer terror and desperate for "help," I turned away from "myself" and in the direction of God.

The rest is history (as relayed in Chapter 1 of this book). Let me be very clear here. The key to my success was not the fact that the Lord guided me to the ultimate diet plan. The real key was the fact that I finally forgot about "myself," asked God for help, and then accepted His help with a promise to spend the rest of my life sharing the secrets He gave me. In other words, after my meltdown, I was touched by God and given a "purpose"—not *just* to rebuild my own health, but to actually forget about my "self"and spend the rest of my life thinking about others. This has made *all* the difference in the world.

So I ask you once again, "Why do *you* want to lose weight and get in shape?" If your reason is related to some temporary gain and is associated with self-centeredness, there is a high likelihood you will fail. But if your true desire is to get in shape, serve others in this world, and fulfill your purpose in life, then, my friend, you have discovered the key to success—and true happiness will never elude you.

Three Keys to Success:

1. BE STILL.
"Be still and know that I am God" (Psalms 46:10). Life is like a game. Dieting is also like a game. But sometimes we are overwhelmed by the game of life. We get confused. We get frustrated. We get too busy. We lose our way. But getting that clarity and direction back doesn't necessarily require you to do something. Actually, sometimes it requires you to do *nothing.* This advice is often thought to be a waste of time. God's reality (as seen in His Word), however, supports that *doing nothing* is one of the great secrets to successful living. And when I say nothing, I mean NOTHING. Sit down somewhere that is quiet and convenient to go to. Sit up straight, close your eyes, and let your mind and thoughts slow down by focusing on your breathing. Don't "think" about it. Breathing is automatic. Instead, just be "aware" of it. Sit quietly for 5-20 minutes, once a day, and notice the positive effect it has on the rest of your life. Be still and be amazed!

2. PRAY.
"The effective fervent prayer of a righteous man avails much" (James 5:16). The second step to success is to ask God, through prayer, what He wants to do with your life. Then let Him guide you. Being in shape is a great goal especially as He desires to use your body to help others here on earth. He will

open every door that you will need to be successful on your diet. The fact that you are reading this book right now is *no* coincidence. God wants you to succeed. He has a plan for you and desires to work through you to fulfill His calling on your life. Your obedience to Him will bring forth many fruits of the spirit—joy, peace, and love. That state of happiness you have been searching for will come by staying connected to the Creator and never taking your eyes off Him. Pray silently each day, and allow the Lord to guide you every step of the way in your life.

> "My *primary* goal in life is to live according to God's will."
> —The Author

3. SET GOALS.

The third key to success is found when you create goals that are not self-centered. In other words, create a list of your goals, and make sure they are not centered solely on you. A goal to get in shape so you can look great and be admired by others is a self-centered goal. A goal to become more *attractive,* for example, so you can share the message of good health and spread the Word of God is a great goal. Do you see the difference? Both goals, when achieved, will produce a more attractive you and place you in the spotlight. Don't follow the self-serving model—take pleasure in doing the things of the Lord. In my life, I have only one purpose—to do God's will. My uncompromising motto is to do His will, His way...all the way. This keeps "me" out of the picture and allows true happiness to shine bright.

As listed above, the three keys to success involve finding your purpose, forgetting about yourself, and then doing God's will, not yours. When I refer to God, I have selected the term I am familiar with and recognize as the Creator of the Universe (the almighty power behind the beauty of creation). You may have your own name and way to describe our beloved Creator. What matters here is that you connect with Him in silence, in prayer, and through His written word.

I am speaking about connecting with God, not about a specific religion. You may be Jewish, Buddhist, Hindu, Zen Buddhist, Catholic, Mormon, or Christian. The form of religion you practice and how you worship God is *your own personal business.* **All roads lead to God for those who put their pride aside and honestly seek Him.** This is not about you; it is about God.

I have experienced many forms of religion: Buddhism, Hinduism, New Age, Zen Buddhism, and Christianity. Each played an important role in helping me "wake up" from the illusion of "self" (ego/pride/desire) to connect with God. (You may read about my spiritual journey in my book entitled *Fit for Christ.* See website for availability.)

Keep in mind, this was *my* path and *my* journey. God truly has a plan for you—keep your heart open to finding it. Your pathway may be completely different than mine. But God, and only God, knows which pathway is best for you. Discover that pathway—ask Him directly through prayer, be "still," and listen for His answer.

"For I know the plans I have for you," declares the Lord, "plans to prosper you and not to harm you, plans to give you a hope and a future."
—Jeremiah 29:11

Chapter 5
The Fat Burning Diet Meal Guidelines

"Nature does her best to teach us. The
more we overeat, the harder she makes it
for us to get close to the table."
—Earl Wilson

LOW-CARB DAYS

In general, you will be avoiding starches, grains, sweet fruits, fruit juice, and anything sweet—except for low-carb fruits—to help deplete liver and muscle glycogen.

Approximate Macronutrient Percentages on Low-Carb Days

30-45% Protein
10-25% Carbohydrate
30-45% Healthy Fats

LOW-CARB FOODS TO CHOOSE FROM:

PROTEIN (acidic):
Chicken, fish, turkey, lean beef, buffalo meat, wild game, low-carb whey protein powder, low-carb soy protein powder, low-fat cottage cheese, cottage cheese, and low-fat cheese.

PROTEIN (neutral to alkaline):
Egg whites, whole eggs, egg white protein powder, nonfat milk, low-fat milk, and grilled chicken breasts.

The Fat Burning Diet

NON-STARCHY VEGETABLES (alkaline):
Artichokes, asparagus, beans (yellow wax or green), bean sprouts, beets, broccoli, cabbage (all varieties), carrots, cauliflower, celery, chives, cucumbers, dandelion greens, eggplant, endive, escarole, garlic, green peas, kale, kohlrabi, leeks, lettuce (all varieties), mustard greens, okra, onions, parsnips, peppers (green, red, jalapeno, Anaheim, etc.), radishes, shallots, spinach, string beans, squash (summer varieties only), Swiss chard, tomatoes, turnips, turnip greens, and watercress.

LOW-CARB FRUITS (alkaline):
(Consume sparingly.)
ALL varieties of fruit *except* bananas, grapes, pears, and dried fruit.

FRIENDLY FATS AND OILS (neutral):
(Use sparingly.)
Olive oil, coconut oil (unrefined), flax seed oil, golden flax seeds, sunflower oil (unrefined), sesame oil (unrefined), fish oils, butter, cream, lecithin (liquid or granules), and avocado.

FRIENDLY FATS AND OILS (alkaline):
(Use sparingly.)
Cream, cheese, almonds, fresh coconut meat from immature (green) coconuts, fresh coconut milk or water from immature (green) coconuts, cream cheese, and sour cream.

FRIENDLY FAT AND OILS (acidic):
(Use sparingly.)
Walnuts, Brazil nuts, macadamia nuts, pecans, filberts (hazelnuts), and pine nuts.

DAIRY PRODUCTS (neutral):
Low-fat cottage cheese, nonfat milk, and low-fat milk.

HIGH-CARB DAYS

In general, you will be consuming a moderate amount of protein along with starches, high-carb fruits, and vegetable juices to load muscle and liver glycogen.

Approximate Macronutrient Percentages on High-Carb Days

15-25% Protein
45-70% Carbohydrate
15-30% Healthy Fats

HIGH-CARB FOODS TO CHOOSE FROM:

STARCHY VEGETABLES (alkaline):
Yams (with skins), sweet potatoes (with skins), corn, corn on the cob, potatoes (with skins), and all varieties of winter squash (butternut, banana, acorn, kabocha, etc.).

PROTEIN (acidic):
(Consume approximately 15-25% of total calories as protein on high-carb days.)
Chicken, fish, turkey, lean beef, buffalo meat, wild game, whey protein powder, low-carb soy protein powder, low-fat cottage cheese, and low-fat cheese.

PROTEIN (alkaline):
(Consume approximately 15-25% of total calories as protein on high-carb days.)
Egg whites, whole eggs, egg white protein powder, chicken breasts, nonfat milk, and low-fat milk.

NON-STARCHY VEGETABLES (alkaline):
Artichokes, asparagus, beans (yellow wax or green), bean sprouts, beets, broccoli, cabbage (all varieties), carrots, cauliflower, celery, chives, cucumbers, dandelion greens, eggplant, endive, escarole, garlic, green peas, kale, kohlrabi, leeks, let-

tuce (all varieties), mustard greens, okra, onions, parsnips, peppers (green, red, jalapeno, Anaheim, etc.), radishes, shallots, spinach, string beans, squash (summer varieties only), Swiss chard, tomatoes, turnips, turnip greens, and watercress.

NOTE: Any of the above vegetables may also be juiced for a special alkaline treat.

HIGH-CARB FRUITS (alkaline):
(Consume no more than 2 pieces or servings daily.)
Bananas, pears, and grapes (1 serving = 12 grapes).

HIGH-CARB DRIED FRUITS (alkaline):
(Consume sparingly.)
Raisins, dates, and figs.

GLUTEN-FREE GRAINS (acidic):
(Choose these only when your body is in an alkaline state.)
Brown rice; rice flour pasta; rice bread (wheat- and gluten-free); corn; corn tortillas; gluten-free, dairy-free, and wheat-free waffles or pancakes; and any whole grain cereal made from millet or rice.

NOTE: Until you pass my wheat and gluten test, listed below, you should avoid wheat, wheat products, oatmeal, rye, barley, and refined grains of all kinds—including most processed breakfast cereals. If you pass the test, then you may occasionally include the grains that contain gluten as listed below. Carbohydrate should still come primarily from alkaline-based vegetable starches (i.e., sweet potatoes, yams, potatoes, and winter squash) instead of from grains (which are acid/mineral-based).

JAY'S WHEAT AND GLUTEN TEST:
Avoid all grains (except rice) for a period of four days. On Day 5, consume whole wheat bread, whole wheat cereal, or whole wheat pancakes for two meals, and note any reactions. If you are sensitive to gluten, you might notice stomach pain, cramp-

ing, gas, bloating, diarrhea, or a messy bowel movement the following day as an outward symptom of gluten intolerance. If you are sensitive to wheat, you may also experience a headache, runny nose, or congestion. If you test for wheat and gluten and no reactions occur, then it should be safe to assume you can consume whole grains occasionally as part of your carbohydrate intake.

GLUTEN-CONTAINING GRAINS (acidic):
(Consume the following only if you passed *Jay's Wheat and Gluten Test* [See page 56] and when your urine is alkaline, as indicated by pH test strips.)

Whole wheat or whole grain bread, whole wheat or whole grain pancakes, whole wheat or whole grain waffles, whole wheat or whole grain pasta, whole wheat berry cereal, cracked wheat cereal, whole wheat cereals that are unsweetened, oatmeal, whole oat cereal, rye bread, barley, and rye cereal.

NATURAL SWEETENERS (neutral):
(Use very sparingly.)
100% pure maple syrup, agave, and xylitol (naturally derived from Birch trees, this natural sweetener is beneficial for preventing dental caries).

DAIRY PRODUCTS (alkaline/neutral):
Sweet dairy whey, low-fat plain yogurt, nonfat plain yogurt, low-fat plain kefir, nonfat milk, and low-fat milk.

DAIRY PRODUCTS (neutral):
(Use very sparingly.)
Butter, cream, and sour cream.

FAT BURNING FATS AND OILS (neutral):
(Use sparingly.)
Olive oil, coconut oil (unrefined), flax seed oil, golden flax seeds, sunflower oil (unrefined), sesame oil (unrefined), fish oils, butter, cream, lecithin (liquid or granules), and avocado.

FRIENDLY FATS AND OILS (alkaline):
(Use sparingly.)
Cream, almonds, fresh coconut meat from immature (green) coconuts, and fresh coconut milk (water) from immature (green) coconuts.

FRIENDLY FATS AND OILS (acidic):
(Use sparingly.)
Walnuts, Brazil nuts, macadamia nuts, pecans, filberts (hazelnuts), and pine nuts.

FOODS AND INGREDIENTS TO AVOID

SUGARS AND SWEET FOODS:
White sugar, sugar, brown sugar, inverted sugar, fructose, high-fructose corn syrup, high-fructose corn sweetener, corn syrup, corn sweetener, dried cane juice, evaporated cane juice, and cane sweeteners.

SUGAR SUBSTITUTES AND SUGAR ALCOHOLS:
Aspartame, sucralose, maltitol, sorbitol, saccharine, and all artificial sweeteners.

ARTIFICIAL FLAVORS AND COLORS (*Read labels carefully!*):
All artificial flavors and colors should be avoided. Soft drinks don't have to be colored and flavored artificially—neither do the foods you consume.

ARTIFICIAL PRESERVATIVES:
BHA, BHT, etc.

CASEIN (A white tasteless, odorless milk and cheese protein used to make plastics, adhesives, paints, and food):
This is a common ingredient in protein bars and protein powders, so beware! Also avoid **calcium caseinate** and **sodium caseinate**.

REFINED FOODS:
White flour, enriched bleached flour, refined oils, processed oils, white flour pancakes, white flour waffles, hydrogenated fats, hydrogenated oils, partially hydrogenated oils, potato chips (fried), corn chips (fried), and tortilla chips.

PROCESSED MEATS:
Assume all packaged, pre-cooked meats are processed, and avoid them—unless they are purchased from a reputable health food store or nutrition center.

CAFFEINE:
The drug caffeine is a bitter white alkaloid derived from coffee, tea, and kola nuts. Caffeine is a stimulant and diuretic, commonly found in caffeinated soft drinks, tea, coffee, and diet pills. Because caffeine is an addictive drug, its consumption should be avoided by choosing decaffeinated tea and coffee and caffeine-free soft drinks.

HOW FOODS AFFECT BLOOD SUGAR LEVELS

Please review the blood sugar charts on the following four pages to gain a clearer understanding of the fat burning process and the problems that can arise when a poor diet is followed.

After reviewing the charts, turn the page and discover more about how to become a fat-melting machine!

> "In the beginner's mind, there are many possibilities, but in the expert's, there are few."
> —Shunryu Suziki

The Fat Burning Diet

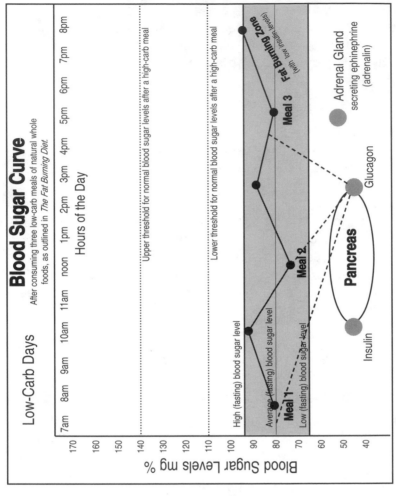

Blood Sugar Curve

After consuming three low-carb meals of natural whole foods, as outlined in *The Fat Burning Diet*.

Low-Carb Days

Hours of the Day

7am 8am 9am 10am 11am noon 1pm 2pm 3pm 4pm 5pm 6pm 7pm 8pm

Blood Sugar Levels mg %

170 160 150 140 130 120 110 100 90 80 70 60 50 40

Upper threshold for normal blood sugar levels after a high-carb meal

Lower threshold for normal blood sugar levels after a high-carb meal

High (fasting) blood sugar level

Average (fasting) blood sugar level

Low (fasting) blood sugar level

Meal 1
Meal 2
Meal 3

Fat Burning Zone (with low insulin levels)

Pancreas

Insulin

Glucagon

Adrenal Gland
secreting ephinephrine (adrenalin)

Low-Carb Days

On low-carb days, insulin is in check because starches and high-carb foods are avoided. This creates very small rises in blood glucose and allows your body to burn fat up to 24 hours a day.

During this time, your pancreas is resting from its job of creating and secreting insulin. Glucagon, the antagonist of insulin, is secreted to lift blood glucose levels instead of lowering them (which is insulin's job). The adrenal glands also get a well-deserved rest because blood sugar levels are in a normal range for the entire period of low-carb eating.

High-Carb Days

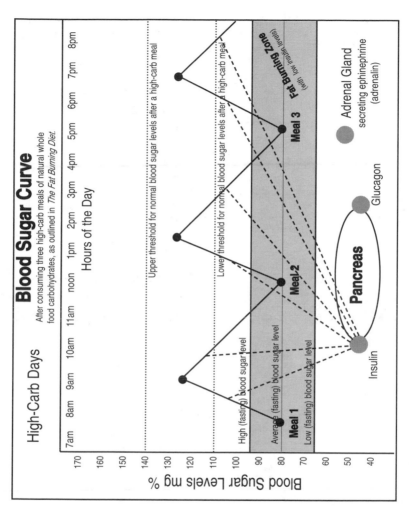

On high-carb days, insulin is produced to manage the blood sugar levels that naturally rise following a high-carb intake.

Insulin is an anabolic hormone that builds muscle, glycogen, and fat. Because low-carb eating precedes high-carb eating, insulin will skip the fat-storing cycle and only assist the body in building muscle tissue and filling glycogen levels.

Because natural carbohydrates are consumed, no sugar or insulin highs or lows are experienced.

61

The Fat Burning Diet

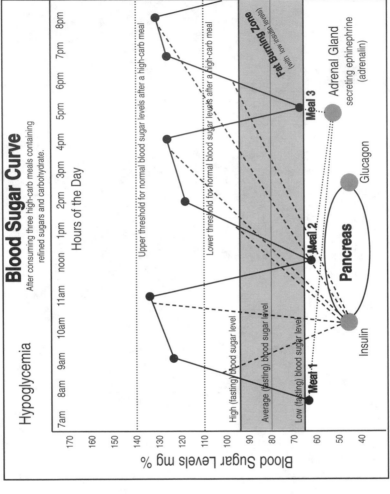

Blood Sugar Curve

After consuming three high-carb meals containing refined sugars and carbohydrate.

Hypoglycemia
(low blood sugar)

Hypoglycemia is directly related to the overindulgence of the wrong type of high-carbohydrate foods—especially refined grains, white flour, sugar, and all refined sweeteners and simple sugars.

Over time, the pancreas can weaken, and insulin receptor sites can fail to recognize insulin, causing surges of insulin to be produced. Delayed insulin production followed by excessive insulin production can cause blood sugar levels and one's moods to become erratic and unstable.

Blood Sugar Curve

After consuming three high-carb meals containing refined sugars and carbohydrate.

Diabetes Type 2

Diabetes Type 2
(hyperglycemia)

If hypoglycemia remains unchecked, it could lead to consistently high blood glucose levels (hyperglycemia). As the pancreas weakens and receptor sites lose their ability to recognize insulin, blood sugar levels can remain high.

High blood sugar levels are actually deadly because glucose in concentration begins to erode the vascular system—especially the tiny vessels in the eyes—which can lead to blindness. The simple solution is to cut back on carbohydrate and to totally avoid refined carbs.

63

The Fat Burning Diet

> "Never eat more than you can lift."
> —Miss Piggy

Chapter 6
The Fat Burning Diet Menu Plans

Below are meal plans for moderately active individuals. At the end of the menu plans, you will find suggestions for modifying the diet if you are highly active, a physical laborer, a diabetic, an endurance athlete, or a bodybuilder.

Don't hesitate to get started. Immediately, jump into the plan, and follow the appropriate menu. DO NOT wait to start the program on a Monday. Dive in NOW, and reap the benefits sooner than later.

The sample daily menus for women contain approximately 1200 to 1600 calories; the sample daily menus for men contain approximately 1600 to 2000 calories. To lose weight effectively, you may need to adjust the number of calories up or down according to your own height, weight, body fat level, activity level, and goals.

NOTE TO VEGETARIANS: If you are avoiding animal flesh, substitute all meat with egg whites, eggs, cottage cheese, protein powder, milk, yogurt, low-fat cheese, tofu, or other forms of vegetarian proteins.

Menus for women start on page 66.
Menus for men start on page 84.

When the term "meditation" is suggested before breakfast on certain days, it means to sit quietly and *be still.*

WOMEN

MONDAY (Low-carb day)

Upon rising: 12 oz water with juice of ½ lemon (or lime) or 1½ tsp acerola berry powder *and* ½ tsp granulated stevia powder.

Exercise 30 minutes first (recommendation).

BREAKFAST

CHOICE #1:
- 16 oz nonfat plain yogurt
- 2 tbs sweet dairy whey
- 1 tsp granulated stevia powder
- 1 medium apple—peeled, cored, and cut into small pieces

Stir ALL ingredients together, and top with 2 tablespoons golden flax seeds (ground fine) or 1 tablespoon chopped raw nuts.

CHOICE #2:
(Protein drink)
- 12 oz pure water
- 3 tbs whey protein or egg white protein, unsweetened and low-carb
- 1 tbs flax seed oil or 2 tbs almond butter
- 6 strawberries, fresh or frozen OK
- 1 tsp granulated stevia powder
- Ice (optional, for a cold drink)

Blend for 15-20 seconds—until creamy smooth.

CHOICE #3:
- Scrambled eggs comprised of 3 egg whites and 1 yolk
- 1 oz cheese (optional)
- 2 celery sticks, 1 steamed zucchini, or 6 strawberries

CHOICE #4:
- 1 low-carb protein bar
- 8 oz nonfat plain yogurt

CHOICE #5:
(Restaurant option)
- 2-3 eggs—cooked, as desired
- Sausage or Canadian bacon

LUNCH

CHOICE #1:
- 3 cups mixed vegetable salad
- 2 tbs salad dressing (low-carb dressings only)
- 3 oz chicken, fish, turkey, or lean beef
- 4 baby carrot sticks

CHOICE #2:
- 1 low-carb protein bar
- 4 cups mixed vegetable salad
- 2 tbs dressing of choice

CHOICE #3:
- 8 oz water mixed with 2 tbs whey or egg white protein
- 4 cups mixed vegetable salad
- 2 tbs dressing of choice

CHOICE #4:
(Restaurant option)
- Grilled salmon or chicken salad
- Dressing on the side
- Small bowl fresh strawberries

The Fat Burning Diet

DINNER

CHOICE #1:
- 2 cups mixed vegetable salad
- 2 tbs salad dressing
- 1 cup steamed broccoli, zucchini, or green beans
- 3 oz chicken, fish, turkey, or lean beef

CHOICE #2:
(Protein drink)
- 12 oz pure water
- 3 tbs whey protein or egg white protein
- 1 tbs flax seed oil or 2 tbs almond butter
- 6 strawberries or ½ cup blueberries, fresh or frozen OK
- 1 tsp stevia powder (optional, for sweetness)
- Ice (optional, for a cold drink)

Blend for 15-20 seconds—until creamy smooth.

CHOICE #3:
(Restaurant option)
- Small steak or medium chicken breast
- Large green salad
- 2 tbs dressing
- Plate of sliced tomatoes

CHOICE #4:
(Restaurant option)
- Grilled chicken or grilled salmon salad
- Dressing on the side
- Small order low-fat cottage cheese

TUESDAY (High-carb day)

Upon rising: 12 oz water with juice of ½ lemon (or lime) or 1½ tsp acerola berry powder *and* ½ tsp granulated stevia powder.

Fifteen minutes of meditation and prayer first.

BREAKFAST

CHOICE #1:
- 16 oz nonfat or low-fat plain yogurt
- 2 tbs sweet dairy whey (feeds lactobacteria in colon)
- 1 apple—peeled, cored, and cut into bite-size pieces
- 2 tbs golden flax seeds (ground fine)

CHOICE #2:
- ¼ large seedless watermelon

CHOICE #3:
- 2 pieces (or servings) fresh fruit

CHOICE #4:
- 16 oz glass fresh vegetable juice

CHOICE #5:
- 2 wheat-free, gluten-free toaster waffles
- 1 pat butter (optional)
- 1 tbs real maple syrup

CHOICE #6:
(Restaurant option)
- 1 order hash brown potatoes or skillet potatoes
- 2 eggs, sunny-side up

The Fat Burning Diet

CHOICE #7:
(Restaurant option—if you are not sensitive to wheat or grains)
- 2 whole grain pancakes
- 1 pat butter
- 1 tbs honey (optional)

LUNCH

CHOICE #1:
- 3 cups mixed vegetable salad
- 2 tbs salad dressing (low-carb dressing only)
- 1 medium-size baked potato, yam, or sweet potato
- 1 pat butter or 1 tbs sour cream
- 2 oz chicken breast

CHOICE #2:
- 1 cup steamed vegetables
- 6 oz steamed or stir-fried tofu
- 1 cup cooked brown rice

CHOICE #3:
(Restaurant option)
- Portion stir-fried vegetables and chicken or tofu
- Portion rice

CHOICE #4:
(Restaurant option)
- Side order corn tortillas
- Side order beans and rice
- Small side guacamole or avocado slices

DINNER

CHOICE #1:
- 2 cups mixed vegetable salad
- 2 tbs salad dressing
- ½ cup cooked pinto beans or black beans
- 1 cup cooked brown rice

CHOICE #2:
- 1 cup baked butternut squash
- 3 cups mixed vegetable salad
- 2 tbs dressing
- 1 hard-boiled egg or 2 oz chicken or turkey

CHOICE #3:
(Complex carbohydrate drink)
- 12 oz pure water
- 2 tbs almond butter or ½ Hass avocado
- 1 tbs whey protein or egg white protein
- 5 tbs dried sweet potato pieces (yam cereal)
- 1 tsp granulated stevia powder

CHOICE #4:
(Restaurant option)
- Portion stir-fried vegetables and tofu
- Portion brown or white rice, cooked or steamed

WEDNESDAY (Low-carb day)

Upon rising: 12 oz water with juice of ½ lemon (or lime) or 1½ tsp acerola berry powder *and* ½ tsp granulated stevia powder.

Exercise 30 minutes.

BREAKFAST

CHOICE #1:
- 16 oz nonfat plain yogurt
- 2 tbs whey protein or egg white protein
- 2 tbs golden flax seeds—ground fine

CHOICE #2:
- 16 oz nonfat plain yogurt
- 2 tbs sweet dairy whey (for feeding lactobacteria)
- 2 tbs golden flax seeds—ground fine
- 1 tsp stevia powder

71

CHOICE #3:
- 1 low-carb protein bar

CHOICE #4:
(On-the-go meal)
- 12 oz water mixed with 3 tbs whey or egg white protein powder
- 1 apple, 1 orange, or 2 tangerines

CHOICE #5:
(Restaurant option)
- Cheese omelet
- Portion low-fat cottage cheese
- Portion tomato slices

LUNCH

CHOICE #1:
- 4 cups mixed vegetable salad
- ½ Hass avocado or 2 tbs low-carb dressing
- 4 oz chicken fish, turkey, or lean beef
- 2 celery sticks

CHOICE #2:
(Fast-food restaurant option)
- Fast-food double burger (no bun)
- Salad bar
- 2 tbs low-carb dressing

CHOICE #3:
- 1 low-carb protein bar
- 2 cups salad
- 1 tbs low-carb dressing

DINNER

CHOICE #1:
- 2 cups steamed zucchini
- 1 oz grated cheese—melt and sprinkle on zucchini
- 3 oz lean beef patty

CHOICE #2:
(Restaurant option)
- Grilled chicken salad
- Dressing on the side (use no more than 2 tbs)
- Lemon wedges (to garnish your water)
- ½ tsp granulated stevia powder (add to lemon water for a sweet taste)

THURSDAY (High-carb day)

Upon rising: 12 oz water with juice of ½ lemon (or lime) or 1½ tsp acerola berry powder *and* ½ tsp granulated stevia powder.

Fifteen minutes of meditation and prayer first.

BREAKFAST

CHOICE #1:
- 16 oz nonfat plain yogurt
- 2 tbs sweet dairy whey
- 1 lactase enzyme (optional, for digesting lactose)
- 1 Navel orange—peeled, sectioned, and cut into pieces
- 1 tsp granulated stevia powder
- 2 tbs golden flax seeds—ground fine
Mix ALL above ingredients in bowl.

CHOICE #2:
- 1 cup cooked rice cereal
- 1 tsp xylitol or 1 tbs pure maple syrup
- 1 banana

CHOICE #3:
- 12 oz low-fat or nonfat milk (use lactose-free milk if you are lactose intolerant)
- 1 tbs whey protein or egg white protein

Mix ingredients together in blender.

CHOICE #4:
(Restaurant option)
- 1 order hash brown potatoes
- 1-2 eggs—cooked, as desired

CHOICE #5:
(On-the-go meal)
- 2-3 pieces (or servings) fresh fruit

LUNCH

CHOICE #1:
- 2 oz tuna or sliced turkey breast
- 1 small yam, baked potato, or sweet potato
- 1 tbs sour cream or 1 pat butter
- 2 cups mixed green salad
- 1 tbs low-fat dressing

CHOICE #2:
(Restaurant option)
- Side order beans and rice
- Side order corn tortillas
- Small side order sliced avocado or fresh guacamole

Skip the chips!

CHOICE #3:
(On-the-go meal)
- 1 banana or 6 baby carrots
- 3 rice crackers, wheat-free and gluten-free
- 2 natural cookies—sugar-free, wheat-free, and gluten-free

DINNER

CHOICE #1:
- 1 cup cooked brown rice
- 3 oz lightly browned tofu or 2 oz grilled chicken
- 1 tbs olive oil (to cook tofu)
- 2 cups steamed peas or mixed vegetables
- 1 tsp Bragg's Liquid Amino (a soy sauce substitute)

CHOICE #2:
(Restaurant option)
- 1 baked potato
- 1 tbs butter, sour cream, or ¼ Hass avocado
- 1 oz cheese or 1 hard-boiled egg (optional, for protein)
- Bacon bits (optional)
- Small dinner salad
- 1 tbs dressing (on the side)

CHOICE #3:
(On-the-go energy drink)
- 16 oz pure water or nonfat milk
- 4 tbs dried sweet potato nuggets or powder
- 1 tbs whey protein or egg white protein
- 1 tsp granulated stevia powder
- 2 tbs golden flax seeds—ground fine
- 1 cup ice cubes (optional, to create an ice cream texture)

Place ALL ingredients in blender, and mix until creamy smooth.

The Fat Burning Diet

FRIDAY (Low-carb day)

Upon rising: 12 oz water with juice of ½ lemon (or lime) or 1½ tsp acerola berry powder *and* ½ tsp granulated stevia powder.

Exercise for 30 minutes.

BREAKFAST

CHOICE #1:
(Protein drink)
- 12 oz pure water
- 3 tbs whey protein or egg white protein (vanilla flavor)
- 1 tbs flax seed oil or 2 tbs golden flax seeds—ground fine
- ½ cup blueberries, fresh or frozen OK
- 1 tsp granulated stevia powder (optional)
- Ice (optional, for a cold drink)

Blend for 15-20 seconds—until creamy smooth.

CHOICE #2:
- 12 oz nonfat or low-fat milk
- 2 tbs whey protein or egg white protein (mix with milk)
- 6 raw almonds or 4 walnut halves

CHOICE #3:
- 2 whole eggs, scrambled
- 5 baby carrots or 3 celery sticks

CHOICE #4:
(On-the-go meal)
- 1 low-carb protein bar
- 8 oz glass nonfat milk or 8 oz nonfat plain yogurt

CHOICE #5:
(Restaurant option)
- Cheese omelet
- Tomato slices, ½ grapefruit, or small bowl of fresh straw-berries

Skip the bread, toast, bagels, and potatoes.

LUNCH

CHOICE #1:
- 3 cups mixed vegetable salad
- 2 tbs salad dressing (low-carb dressings only)
- 3 oz chicken, fish, turkey, or lean beef
- 4 baby carrot sticks

CHOICE #2:
Protein drink—same as today's breakfast drink, CHOICE #1

CHOICE #3:
(Restaurant option)
- Stir-fried vegetables with chicken

Skip the rice.

CHOICE #4:
- 1 low-carb protein bar
- 6 baby carrots

DINNER

CHOICE #1:
- 2 cups mixed vegetable salad
- 2 tbs salad dressing
- 1 cup steamed broccoli, zucchini, or green beans
- 3 oz chicken, fish, turkey, or lean beef
- 1 glass limeade (12 oz water, juice ½ lime, and ¼ tsp ste-via powder)

CHOICE #2:
LOW-CARB PIZZA
- 2 whole eggs (whipped and cooked like flat omelet)
- 3 tbs pizza sauce
- 1 oz mozzarella cheese

Cook eggs into flat omelet, and slide onto plate. Top with pizza sauce and cheese. Warm in toaster oven or microwave until cheese melts. Enjoy!

CHOICE #3:
(Restaurant or home option)
CHEF SALAD
- 4 cups mixed vegetable salad
- 1 hard-boiled egg—peeled and chopped
- 1 oz chopped turkey or chicken breast
- 1 oz low-fat cheese
- 2 tbs dressing of choice

CHOICE #4:
(Restaurant option)
- Small steak
- Large green salad
- Dressing on the side (use sparingly)
- Steamed vegetables

Avoid bread if they offer it.

CHOICE #5:
(Restaurant option)
- Grilled chicken Caesar salad
- Small bowl cherry tomatoes or tomato slices

SATURDAY (High-carb day and FREE meal night)

Upon rising: 12 oz water with juice of ½ lemon (or lime) or 1½ tsp acerola berry powder *and* ½ tsp granulated stevia powder.

Fifteen minutes of meditation and prayer first.

BREAKFAST

CHOICE #1:
- 2 wheat-free, gluten-free toaster waffles
- 1 pat butter or 1 tbs raw almond butter
- 1 tbs REAL maple syrup
- 1 egg—cooked, as desired

CHOICE #2:
- 2 wheat-free, gluten-free pancakes
- 1 pat butter
- 1 tbs REAL maple syrup
- 1 egg—cooked, as desired

CHOICE #3:
- 16 oz nonfat plain yogurt
- 2 tbs sweet dairy whey
- 1 lactase enzyme (optional, for digesting lactose)
- 1 small sliced banana or 8 grapes

CHOICE #4:
(Restaurant option)
- 2 whole grain pancakes (eat only if you are not wheat-, gluten-, or grain-sensitive)
- 1 pat real butter (not margarine!)
- 1 tbs REAL maple syrup or honey

CHOICE #5:
(Restaurant option)
- 1 cup cooked oatmeal (eat only if you are not gluten- or grain-sensitive)
- 1 tsp granulated stevia powder
- 3 tbs raisins
- 1 banana

CHOICE #6:
- 1 small cantaloupe

CHOICE #7:
- 2-3 pieces (or servings) fresh fruit

CHOICE #8:
- 12 oz glass fresh vegetable juice

LUNCH

CHOICE #1:
- 1 cup wheat-free, gluten-free pasta, cooked
- 3 tbs low-fat pasta sauce
- 2 cups mixed green salad
- 1 tbs dressing
- 2 oz turkey or chicken breast

CHOICE #2:
SWEET POTATO MILKSHAKE
- 12 oz nonfat milk (lactose-free if you are lactose intolerant)
- 5 tbs dried sweet potato pieces
- 1 tbs raw almond butter

Mix in blender—until creamy smooth.

CHOICE #3:
- 1 small baked yam or sweet potato
- 1 pat butter or 4 slices avocado
- 2 oz sliced turkey breast

CHOICE #4:
- 1 cup cooked corn
- 4 oz tofu
- ½ cup cooked brown rice

CHOICE #5:
(Restaurant option)
- Stir-fried vegetables with tofu, chicken, fish, or beef
- Portion brown or white rice, cooked or steamed

CHOICE #6:
(Restaurant option)
- 1 bean tostada or chicken enchilada
- Portion brown or white rice, cooked or steamed

DINNER (FREE MEAL)

It's time to party!

"ANYTHING GOES" for one full hour of culinary ecstasy! Pizza, pasta, lasagna, steak, fried chicken, seafood, lobster, cookies, pie, ice cream, donuts, and bread are all on the menu, so go for it, and enjoy! You must time this meal and limit it to only 60 minutes. No cheating.

SUNDAY (Low-carb breakfast and lunch; high-carb dinner)

Upon rising: 12 oz water with juice of ½ lemon (or lime) or 1½ tsp acerola berry powder *and* ½ tsp granulated stevia powder.

BREAKFAST

CHOICE #1:
- Two-egg omelet topped with 1 oz cheese
- 2 celery sticks filled with 1 tbs almond butter or 1 small sliced tomato

CHOICE #2:
(Protein drink)
- 16 oz pure water or nonfat milk
- 3 tbs whey protein or egg white protein (flavor of choice)
- 1 tbs sour cream or 2 tbs golden flax seeds—ground fine
- 1 tsp granulated stevia powder

Mix in blender for 15-30 seconds.

CHOICE #3:
(Restaurant option)
- 1 grapefruit—cut in half, sectioned, and sprinkled with stevia powder
- 2 eggs—cooked, as desired

CHOICE #4:
(Restaurant option)
- 1 lean beef patty or chicken breast
- 1 small dish low-fat cottage cheese
- 1 small dish fresh strawberries or 1 sliced tomato

CHOICE #5:
- 16 oz nonfat plain yogurt
- 2 tbs sweet dairy whey
- 1 lactase enzyme (optional, for digesting lactose)
- 1 tsp granulated stevia powder
- 4 raw walnut halves

Mix ALL ingredients in bowl, and enjoy!

LUNCH

CHOICE #1:
- 3 cups mixed vegetable salad
- 1 tbs dressing
- 3 oz water-packed tuna
- 1 oz grated cheese

CHOICE #2:
- 2 cups steamed green beans
- 3 oz deli-sliced turkey, chopped
- 5 raw almonds, chopped

Top with squirt of mustard and serve.

CHOICE #3:
(Restaurant option)
- 3 oz grilled fish
- 1 cup steamed vegetables
- Small salad
- Dressing on the side

CHOICE #4:
(Restaurant option)
- Grilled chicken Caesar salad

DINNER (FREE MEAL)

CHOICE #1:
- 1 cup wheat-free, gluten-free pasta, cooked
- 3 tbs pasta sauce
- 1 cup steamed zucchini
- 2 oz chicken, fish, or beef *or* 1 oz cheese

CHOICE #2:
- ½ cup pinto or black beans, cooked
- ½ cup brown rice, cooked
- 2 corn tortillas
- 2 tbs fresh salsa or ½ small tomato, chopped
- 2 oz baked corn chips

Roll beans and rice inside tortillas. Top with salsa.

CHOICE #3:
(Restaurant option)
- 1 fish taco
- 1 bean tostada
- Portion brown or white rice, cooked or steamed

CHOICE #4:
(Restaurant option)
- Soup of the day
- Baked potato
- 1 pat butter
- Small dinner salad
- Dressing on the side

CHOICE #5:
(Restaurant option)
- Chicken or tofu and snow peas, stir-fried
- Portion brown or white rice, cooked or steamed

MEN

MONDAY (Low-carb day)

Upon rising: 12 oz water with juice of ½ lemon (or lime) or 1½ tsp acerola berry powder *and* ½ tsp granulated stevia powder.

Exercise 30 minutes first (recommendation).

BREAKFAST

CHOICE #1:
- 24 oz nonfat plain yogurt
- 3 tbs sweet dairy whey
- 1 tsp granulated stevia powder
- 1 large apple—peeled, cored, and cut into small pieces

Stir ALL the above ingredients together in bowl, and top with 2 tablespoons finely ground golden flax seeds.

CHOICE #2:
(Protein drink)
- 12 oz pure water
- 4 tbs whey protein or egg white protein (vanilla flavor)
- 1 tbs flax seed oil or 2 tbs golden flax seeds, ground fine
- 8 strawberries, fresh or frozen OK
- 1 tsp granulated stevia powder
- Ice (optional, for a cold drink)

Blend for 15-20 seconds—until creamy smooth.

CHOICE #3:
- Scrambled eggs made with 5 egg whites and 2 yolks
- 1 oz cheese
- 3 celery sticks, 1 apple, or 8 strawberries

CHOICE #4:
- 1 low-carb protein bar
- 8 oz nonfat plain yogurt mixed with 1 tbs whey or egg white protein

CHOICE #5:
(Restaurant option)
- 4 eggs—cooked, as desired
- 1 order sausage or Canadian bacon

LUNCH

CHOICE #1:
- 4 cups mixed vegetable salad
- 2 tbs salad dressing (low-carb dressings only)
- 5 oz chicken, fish, turkey, or lean beef
- 4 baby carrot sticks

CHOICE #2:
- 1-2 low-carb protein bars
- 4 cups mixed vegetable salad
- 2 tbs dressing of choice

CHOICE #3:
- 12 oz water mixed with 3 tbs whey protein or egg white protein
- 4 cups mixed vegetable salad
- 2 tbs dressing of choice

CHOICE #4:
(Restaurant option)
- Grilled salmon or chicken salad
- Dressing on the side
- Small bowl fresh strawberries or sliced tomatoes

DINNER

CHOICE #1:
- 4 cups mixed vegetable salad
- 3 tbs salad dressing
- 1 cup steamed broccoli, zucchini, or green beans
- 6 oz chicken, fish, turkey, or lean beef

CHOICE #2:
(Protein drink)
- 16 oz pure water
- 4 tbs whey protein or egg white protein (vanilla flavor)
- 1 tbs flax seed oil or 2 tbs golden flax seeds—ground fine
- ½ cup blueberries or 6 strawberries, fresh or frozen OK
- 1 tsp granulated stevia powder
- Ice (optional, for a cold drink)
Blend for 15-20 seconds—until creamy smooth.

CHOICE #3:
(Restaurant option)
- Medium-size steak or chicken breast
- Large green salad
- 2 tbs dressing
- Plate sliced tomatoes

CHOICE #4:
(Restaurant option)
- Grilled chicken or grilled salmon salad
- Dressing on the side
- Small order low-fat cottage cheese

TUESDAY (High-carb day)

Upon rising: 12 oz water with juice of ½ lemon (or lime) or 1½ tsp acerola berry powder *and* ½ tsp granulated stevia powder.

Fifteen minutes of meditation and prayer first.

BREAKFAST

CHOICE #1:
- 24 oz nonfat or low-fat plain yogurt
- 2 tbs sweet dairy whey (for feeding lactobacteria)
- 1 apple—peeled, cored, and cut into bite-size pieces
- 2 tbs golden flax seeds, ground fine

CHOICE #2:
- ½ large seedless watermelon

CHOICE #3:
- 2-4 pieces (or servings) fresh fruit

CHOICE #4:
- 16 oz glass fresh vegetable juice

CHOICE #5:
- 3 wheat-free, gluten-free toaster waffles
- 1 pat butter (optional)
- 1 tbs REAL maple syrup
- 2-3 eggs—cooked, as desired

The Fat Burning Diet

CHOICE #6:
(Restaurant option)
- 2 orders hash brown potatoes or skillet potatoes
- 3 eggs sunny-side up

CHOICE #7:
(Restaurant option—if you are not sensitive to wheat or grains)
- 3 whole grain pancakes
- 1 pat butter
- 1 tbs honey (optional)

LUNCH

CHOICE #1:
- 4 cups mixed vegetable salad
- 2 tbs salad dressing (very low-carb dressing only)
- 1 large baked potato, yam, or sweet potato
- 1 pat butter or 1 tbs sour cream
- 2 oz chicken breast

CHOICE #2:
- 1 cup steamed vegetables
- 6 oz steamed or stir-fried tofu
- 1½ cup cooked brown rice

CHOICE #3:
(Restaurant option)
- Stir-fried vegetables *and* chicken or tofu
- Portion brown or white rice, cooked or steamed

CHOICE #4:
(Restaurant option)
- Side order corn tortillas (3-4)
- Side order beans and rice
- Side order guacamole or avocado slices

DINNER

CHOICE #1:
- 2 cups mixed vegetable salad
- 2 tbs salad dressing
- ½ cup cooked pinto beans or black beans
- 2 cups cooked brown rice

CHOICE #2:
- 1½ cups baked butternut squash
- 3 cups mixed vegetable salad
- 2 tbs dressing
- 2 hard-boiled eggs or 2 oz chicken or turkey

CHOICE #3:
(Complex carbohydrate drink)
- 24 oz pure water or nonfat milk
- 2 tbs golden flax seeds—ground fine
- 1 tbs whey protein or egg white protein (vanilla flavor)
- 6 tbs dried sweet potato nuggets or powder
- 1 tsp granulated stevia powder

Mix ALL ingredients in blender for 25-40 seconds.

CHOICE #4:
(Restaurant option)
- Stir-fried vegetables and tofu or chicken
- Portion brown or white rice, cooked or steamed

WEDNESDAY (Low-carb day)

Upon rising: 12 oz water with juice of ½ lemon (or lime) or 1½ tsp acerola berry powder *and* ½ tsp granulated stevia powder.

Exercise 30 minutes first.

BREAKFAST

CHOICE #1:
- 16 oz nonfat plain yogurt
- 2 tbs whey protein or egg white protein (flavor of choice)
- 2 tbs golden flax seeds—ground fine

CHOICE #2:
- 24 oz nonfat plain yogurt
- 2 tbs sweet dairy whey (for feeding lactobacteria)
- 1 lactase enzyme (optional, for digesting lactose)
- 1 tsp granulated stevia powder

CHOICE #3:
- 1-2 low-carb protein bars

CHOICE #4:
(On-the-go meal)
- 16 oz water mixed with 4 tbs whey protein or egg white protein powder (flavor of choice)
- 1 apple, 1 orange, or 2 tangerines

CHOICE #5:
(Restaurant option)
- Cheese omelet
- Low-fat cottage cheese
- Tomato slices

LUNCH

CHOICE #1:
- 4 cups mixed vegetable salad
- ½ Hass avocado or 2 tbs low-carb dressing
- 6 oz chicken fish, turkey, or lean beef
- 2 celery sticks or 4 baby carrots

CHOICE #2:
(Fast-food restaurant option)
- Fast-food double burger (no bun)
- Salad bar
- 2 tbs low-carb dressing
- 1 oz cheese (optional)

CHOICE #3:
- 1-2 low-carb protein bars
- 2 cups salad
- 1 tbs low-carb dressing

DINNER

CHOICE #1:
- 2 cups steamed zucchini
- 2 oz grated cheese (top the zucchini)
- 6 oz lean beef patty

CHOICE #2:
(Restaurant option)
- Grilled chicken salad
- Dressing on the side (use no more than 2 tbs)
- Lemon wedges (to garnish your water)
- 1 tsp granulated stevia powder (add to lemon water for a sweet taste)

The Fat Burning Diet

THURSDAY (High-carb day)

Upon rising: 12 oz water with juice of ½ lemon (or lime) or 1½ tsp acerola berry powder *and* ½ tsp granulated stevia powder.

15 minutes of meditation and prayer first.

BREAKFAST

CHOICE #1:
- 24 oz nonfat plain yogurt
- 2 tbs sweet dairy whey
- 1 lactase enzyme (optional, for digesting lactose)
- 1 Navel orange—peeled, sectioned, and cut into small pieces
- 1 tsp granulated stevia powder
- 2 tbs golden flax seeds—ground fine

Mix ALL ingredients in bowl.

CHOICE #2:
- 2 cups cooked rice cereal
- 2 tsp xylitol or 1 tbs pure maple syrup
- 1 banana
- 1-2 eggs—cooked, as desired

CHOICE #3:
- 16 oz low-fat or nonfat milk (use lactose-free milk if you are lactose intolerant)
- 1 tbs whey protein or egg white protein (flavor of choice)

Mix together in blender.

CHOICE #4:
(Restaurant option)
- 2 orders hash brown potatoes
- 2-3 eggs—cooked, as desired

CHOICE #5:
(On-the-go meal)
- 2-4 pieces (or servings) fresh fruit

LUNCH

CHOICE #1
- 2 oz tuna or sliced turkey breast
- 1 large yam, baked potato, or sweet potato
- 1 tbs sour cream or 1 pat butter
- 2 cups mixed green salad
- 1 tbs low-fat dressing

CHOICE #2:
(Restaurant option)
- Side order beans and rice
- Side order corn tortillas
- Small side order sliced avocado or guacamole
Skip the chips!

CHOICE #3:
(On-the-go meal)
- 2 bananas or 10 baby carrots
- 4 rice crackers, wheat-free and gluten-free
- 1 natural cookie—sugar-free, wheat-free, and gluten-free

DINNER

CHOICE #1:
- 1½ cups cooked brown rice
- 6 oz lightly browned tofu or 2 oz grilled chicken
- 1 tbs olive oil (to cook tofu)
- 1 cup steamed peas or mixed vegetables
- 1 tsp Bragg's Liquid Aminos (a soy sauce substitute)

The Fat Burning Diet

CHOICE #2:
(Restaurant option)
- 1 large baked potato
- 1 tbs butter or sour cream or ¼ Hass avocado
- 1 oz cheese or 1 hard-boiled egg
- Bacon bits
- Small dinner salad
- 1 tbs dressing (on the side)

CHOICE #3:
(On-the-go energy drink)
- 12 oz pure water
- 7 tbs dried sweet potato nuggets
- 2 tbs whey protein or egg white protein (vanilla flavor)
- 1 tsp granulated stevia powder
- ½ peeled and pitted Hass avocado or 2 tbs almond butter
- 1 cup ice cubes (optional, to create an ice cream texture)

Place ALL ingredients in blender, and mix until creamy smooth.

FRIDAY (Low-carb day)

Upon rising: 12 oz water with juice of ½ lemon (or lime) or 1½ tsp acerola berry powder *and* ½ tsp granulated stevia powder.

Exercise for 30 minutes first.

BREAKFAST

CHOICE #1:
(Protein drink)
- 12 oz pure water
- 4 tbs whey protein or egg white protein (vanilla flavor)
- 1 tbs flax seed oil or 2 tbs golden flax seeds—ground fine
- ½ cup blueberries, fresh or frozen OK
- 1 tsp granulated stevia powder (optional)
- Ice (optional, for a cold drink)

Blend for 15-20 seconds—until creamy smooth.

CHOICE #2:
- 16 oz nonfat or low-fat milk (use lactose-free milk if you are lactose intolerant)
- 3 tbs whey protein or egg white protein (vanilla flavor)—mix with milk
- 6 raw almonds or 4 walnut halves

CHOICE #3:
(On-the-go meal)
- 1 low-carb protein bar
- 12 oz glass nonfat milk or 12 oz nonfat plain yogurt

CHOICE #4:
(Restaurant option)
- Large cheese omelet *or* cheese and meat omelet
- Tomato slices, ½ grapefruit, or small bowl fresh strawberries
- Small dish low-fat cottage cheese

Skip the bread, toast, bagels, and potatoes.

LUNCH

CHOICE #1:
- 4 cups mixed vegetable salad
- 2 tbs salad dressing (low-carb dressings only)
- 6 oz chicken, fish, turkey, or lean beef
- 4 baby carrot sticks

CHOICE #2:
Protein drink—same as today's breakfast drink, CHOICE #1

CHOICE #3:
(Restaurant option)
- Stir-fried vegetables with chicken

Skip the rice.

CHOICE #4:
- 1-2 low-carb protein bars
- 6 baby carrots

DINNER

CHOICE #1:
- 4 cups mixed vegetable salad
- 2 tbs salad dressing
- 1 cup steamed broccoli, zucchini, or green beans
- 6 oz chicken, fish, turkey, or lean beef
- 1 glass limeade (12 oz water, juice of ½ lime, and ¼ tsp stevia powder)

CHOICE #2:
LOW-CARB PIZZA
- 4 whole eggs—whipped and cooked like flat omelet
- 4 tbs pizza sauce
- 2-3 oz mozzarella cheese
- Top with 2 oz chicken, fish, turkey, or beef (optional)

Cook eggs as flat omelet, and slide onto plate. Top with pizza sauce and cheese. Warm in toaster oven, or microwave until cheese melts. Enjoy!

CHOICE #3:
(Restaurant or home option)
CHEF SALAD
- 4 cups mixed vegetable salad
- 1 hard-boiled egg, peeled and chopped
- 3 oz chopped turkey or chicken breast
- 2 oz low-fat cheese
- 2 tbs dressing of choice

CHOICE #4:
(Restaurant option)
- Medium-size steak
- Large green salad
- Dressing on the side (use sparingly)
- Steamed vegetables

Avoid warm bread if they offer it.

CHOICE #5:
(Restaurant option)
- Grilled chicken Caesar salad
- Small bowl cherry tomatoes or tomato slices

SATURDAY (High-carb day and FREE MEAL night!)

Upon rising: 12 oz water with juice of ½ lemon (or lime) or 1½ tsp acerola berry powder *and* ½ tsp granulated stevia powder.

Fifteen minutes of meditation and prayer first.

BREAKFAST

CHOICE #1:
- 3-4 wheat-free, gluten-free toaster waffles
- 1 pat butter or 1 tbs raw almond butter
- 1 tbs REAL maple syrup
- 1-2 eggs—cooked, as desired

CHOICE #2:
- 3 wheat-free, gluten-free pancakes
- 1 pat butter
- 1 tbs REAL maple syrup
- 1-2 eggs—cooked, as desired

CHOICE #3:
- 24 oz nonfat plain yogurt
- 2 tbs sweet dairy whey
- 1 lactase enzyme (optional, for digesting lactose)
- 1 sliced banana or 8 grapes
- 1-2 wheat-free, gluten-free toaster waffles (optional)

CHOICE #4:
(Restaurant option)
- 3 whole grain pancakes (eat only if you are not wheat-, gluten-, or grain-sensitive)
- 1 pat real butter (not margarine!)
- 1 tbs pure maple syrup or honey
- 1-2 eggs—cooked, as desired

CHOICE #5:
(Restaurant option)
- 2 cups cooked oatmeal (eat only if you are not gluten- or grain-sensitive)
- 1 tsp granulated stevia powder (optional)
- 3 tbs raisins
- 1 banana

CHOICE #6:
- 1 cantaloupe

CHOICE #7:
- 2-4 pieces (or servings) fresh fruit

CHOICE #8:
- 16 oz glass fresh vegetable juice

LUNCH

CHOICE #1:
- 1½ cups wheat- and gluten-free pasta, cooked
- 3 tbs low-fat pasta sauce
- 2 cups mixed green salad
- 1 tbs dressing
- 2 oz turkey or chicken breast

CHOICE #2:
SWEET POTATO MILKSHAKE
- 16 oz nonfat milk (lactose-free if you are lactose intolerant)
- 5 tbs dried sweet potato cereal (yam nuggets)
- 1 tbs raw almond butter

Mix in blender—until creamy smooth.

CHOICE #3:
- 1 baked yam or sweet potato
- 1 pat butter or a few slices of avocado
- 2 oz sliced turkey breast

CHOICE #4:
- 1 cup cooked corn
- 6 oz tofu—browned in skillet
- 2 cups cooked brown rice

CHOICE #5:
(Restaurant option)
- Stir-fried vegetables with tofu, chicken, fish, or beef
- Portion brown or white rice, cooked or steamed

CHOICE #6:
(Restaurant option)
- 2 bean tostadas
- 1 chicken enchilada or taco
- Portion brown or white rice, cooked or steamed

The Fat Burning Diet

DINNER (FREE MEAL)

It's time to party!

"ANYTHING GOES" for one full hour of culinary ecstasy! Pizza, pasta, lasagna, steak, fried chicken, seafood, lobster, cookies, pie, ice cream, donuts, and bread are all on the menu. Go for it, and enjoy! You must time this meal and limit it to 60 minutes. No cheating.

SUNDAY (Low-carb breakfast and lunch; high-carb dinner)

Upon rising: 12 oz water with juice of ½ lemon (or lime) or 1½ tsp acerola berry powder *and* ½ tsp granulated stevia powder.

BREAKFAST

CHOICE #1:
- 3-egg omelet topped with 1 oz cheese
- 2 celery sticks filled with 1 tbs almond butter
- 3 oz low-fat cottage cheese
- 1 tomato, sliced

CHOICE #2:
(Protein drink)
- 16 oz pure water or nonfat milk
- 3 tbs whey protein or egg white protein (flavor of choice)
- 1 tbs sour cream or 1 tbs raw almond butter
- 1 tsp granulated stevia powder
Mix in blender for 15-30 seconds.

CHOICE #3:
(Restaurant option)
- 1 grapefruit—halved, sectioned, and sprinkled with granulated stevia powder
- 4 eggs or large omelet of choice—cooked, as desired

CHOICE #4:
(Restaurant option)
- 1 lean beef patty or chicken breast
- 1 small dish low-fat cottage cheese
- 1 small dish fresh strawberries or 1 tomato, sliced

CHOICE #5:
(Colon support)
- 24 oz nonfat plain yogurt
- 2 tbs sweet dairy whey
- 1 lactase enzyme (optional, for digesting lactose)
- 1 tsp granulated stevia powder
- 2 tbs golden flax seeds—ground fine

Mix ALL ingredients in bowl, and enjoy.

LUNCH

CHOICE #1:
- 4 cups mixed vegetable salad
- 2 tbs dressing
- 6 oz water-packed tuna
- 1-2 oz grated cheese or ½ avocado

CHOICE #2:
- 2 cups steamed green beans
- 6 oz deli-sliced turkey, chopped
- 8 raw almonds, chopped
- Top with squirt or 2 of mustard

CHOICE #3:
(Restaurant option)
- 6 oz grilled fish
- 1 cup steamed vegetables
- Large salad dressing on the side

CHOICE #4:
(Restaurant option)
- Grilled chicken Caesar salad

DINNER

CHOICE #1:
- 1½ cups cooked wheat-free, gluten-free pasta
- 4 tbs pasta sauce
- 1 cup steamed zucchini
- 2 oz chicken, fish, or beef *or* 1 oz cheese

CHOICE #2:
- ½ cup pinto or black beans, cooked
- 1 cup brown rice, cooked
- 3-5 corn tortillas
- 2 tbs fresh salsa or ½ small tomato, chopped
- 2 oz baked corn chips

Roll beans and rice inside tortillas, and top with salsa.

CHOICE #3:
(Restaurant option)
- 1 fish taco
- 2 bean tostadas
- Portion rice

CHOICE #4:
(Restaurant option)
- Soup of the day
- 1 baked potato
- 1 pat butter
- Large dinner salad
- Dressing on the side

CHOICE #5:
(Restaurant option)
- Portion chicken or tofu and snow peas, stir-fried
- Portion brown or white rice, cooked or steamed

As you can see, The Fat Burning Diet is the ultimate way to eat. You get it all and can gain energy and lose weight in the process.

The Fat Burning Diet, as listed above, is for a moderately active individual. Activity is critical to good health. You should try to exercise at least 30 minutes a session, three to four days a week.

It is simple and easy to adjust The Fat Burning Diet to meet your individual needs. If you are active to the point that you burn away glycogen faster than the every-other-day cycle (of the original plan), then you simply increase the carbohydrate portions of the meals on carb-loading days. If your activity level should decrease at any time, simply cut back slightly on the carbohydrate portions on your carb-loading days. It's that easy!

On The Fat Burning Diet, you are never deprived and can lose excess weight almost without effort.

Fear knocked at the door.
Faith answered.
No one was there.
—Unknown

Chapter 7
Table of Food Composition

ABBREVIATIONS:

Amount = Amt
Calories = Cal
Carbohydrate = Carb
Grams = g
Ounce = oz
Quart = qt
Protein = Prot
Teaspoon = tsp
Tablespoon = tbs

Note: All meats listed in the following charts are broiled, roasted, or baked—not fried. All amounts listed are approximations.

FOOD GROUP I

PROTEIN FOODS	Amt	Cal	Prot/g	Carb/g	Fat/g
Beef, extra lean ground	4 oz	265	28	0	16
Beef, lean ground	3 oz	240	24	0	15
Beef round steak	7 oz	470	52	0	27
Beef sirloin, choice	4 oz	320	32	0	21
Beef, T-bone steak	4 oz	322	26	0	23
Chicken breast	3 oz	198	29	0	8
Chicken meat, skinless	4 oz	215	33	0	9
Chicken thigh, skinless	4 oz	216	27	0	11
Deer/venison	4 oz	178	34	0	4
Egg, large/whole	1 ea	75	6	0	5
Egg white, cooked	1 ea	17	4	0	0

The Fat Burning Diet

Egg yolk, cooked	1 ea	59	3	0	5
Ocean perch	5 oz	128	24	0	2
Swordfish	4 oz	164	27	0	6
Tuna, water-packed	4 oz	120	28	0	2
Turkey, dark/skinless	4 oz	210	32	0	8
Turkey, light/skinless	4 oz	160	34	0	2
Turkey patty, ground	2 oz	194	23	0	11

FOOD GROUP II

VEGETABLES	Amt	Cal	Prot/g	Carb/g	Fat/g
Asparagus spears	6 ea	20	2	4	0
Broccoli, raw	4 oz	32	4	6	0
Brussels sprouts, raw	4 oz	49	4	10	0
Butter lettuce	1 ea	45	4	9	1
Cabbage, raw	4 oz	28	2	6	0
Carrots, raw	1 ea	31	1	7	0
Cauliflower, raw	4 oz	28	2	6	0
Celery, raw	4 oz	18	1	4	0
Chili peppers, hot red	1 oz	11	1	3	0
Collards, raw	4 oz	35	2	8	0
Corn on cob, boiled	1 ea	71	3	17	1
Cucumber slices	1 oz	3	0	0	0
Dandelion greens, raw	4 oz	51	3	10	1
Escarole, raw	4 oz	19	2	4	0
Green bell peppers	1 oz	8	0	2	0
Green peas, raw	4 oz	190	12	35	1
Iceberg lettuce, raw	2 oz	5	0	1	1
Kale, raw	4 oz	57	4	11	1
Kohlrabi, raw	4 oz	25	2	6	0
Mustard greens, raw	4 oz	30	3	6	0
Onions, raw	4 oz	43	2	10	0
Parsley, chopped/raw	1 tbs	1	0	0	0
Parsnips, raw/sliced	1 tbs	6	0	2	0
Radishes, red/raw	4 ea	3	0	1	0
Romaine lettuce, raw	1 oz	3	0	1	0
Spinach, raw	4 oz	25	3	4	0
Summer squash, raw	8 oz	20	1	6	0
Tomato, medium/raw	1 ea	26	1	6	0

FOOD GROUP III

FRESH FRUIT	Amt	Cal	Prot/g	Carb/g	Fat/g
Apples, medium	1 ea	81	0	21	0
Applesauce, unswtnd.	4 oz	48	0	13	0
Apricots, pitted	3 ea	51	2	12	0

	Amt	Cal	Prot/g	Carb/g	Fat/g
Avocados, raw	6 oz	306	4	12	30
Bananas, medium/raw	4 oz	104	1	26	1
Blackberries, raw	8 oz	118	2	29	1
Blueberries, raw	8 oz	127	2	32	1
Cantaloupe, raw	12 oz	119	3	29	1
Grapefruits, medium	1 ea	37	1	9	1
Grapes, raw	8 oz	53	1	12	1
Honeydew, raw	12 oz	99	1	26	0
Kiwifruit, raw	1 ea	46	1	11	0
Mangos, medium/raw	0 ea	67	1	18	0
Oranges, medium/raw	1 ea	62	1	16	0
Peaches, medium	1 ea	37	1	10	1
Pears, medium	1 ea	98	1	25	1
Pineapples, raw	8 oz	111	1	28	1
Plums, medium	1 ea	36	1	9	0
Prunes, dried	4 oz	270	3	71	1
Red raspberries, raw	8 oz	111	2	26	1
Strawberries, raw	8 oz	68	1	16	1
Watermelons, 6"x 2" slice	1 ea	170	3	40	1

FOOD GROUP IV

FATS AND OILS	Amt	Cal	Prot/g	Carb/g	Fat/g
Almonds, raw	4 oz	668	23	23	60
Brazil nuts, raw	4 oz	744	17	15	76
Butter	1 tbs	102	0	0	12
Canola oil	1 tbs	120	0	0	13
Cashews	1 oz	163	5	9	13
Coconut, dried	4 tbs	129	2	5	13
English walnuts, raw	10 ea	130	3	4	12
Flax seed oil	1 tbs	128	0	0	14
Macadamia nuts	1 oz	199	3	4	21
Mixed nuts, roasted	1 oz	168	5	7	15
Olive oil	1 tbs	119	0	0	14
Peanuts, dry-roasted	4 oz	663	27	24	56
Pecan halves, raw	1 oz	189	2	5	19
Pine nuts, raw	1 oz	146	7	4	14
Pistachio nuts, raw	4 oz	655	23	28	55
Pumpkin seeds, raw	1 oz	126	5	15	5
Safflower oil	1 tbs	120	0	0	14
Sesame seeds, raw	1 oz	162	5	7	14
Sunflower seeds, raw	1 oz	161	7	5	14
Wheat germ oil	1 tbs	120	0	0	14

The Fat Burning Diet

<u>FOOD GROUP V</u>

DAIRY PRODUCTS	Amt	Cal	Prot/g	Carb/g	Fat/g
Blue cheese	1 oz	100	6	1	8
Cheddar cheese	1 oz	114	7	0	9
Colby cheese	1 oz	111	7	1	9
Cottage cheese (reg)	8 oz	233	28	6	10
Cream cheese	1 oz	99	2	1	10
Half-and-half cream	1 tbs	20	1	1	2
Sour cream	1 tbs	31	1	1	3
Soy milk, plain	8 oz	75	6	4	4
Whipping cream	1 tbs	51	0	1	6
Whole milk	8 oz	138	8	11	8
Yogurt, nonfat/plain	8 oz	126	13	17	0
Yogurt, whole/plain	8 oz	139	8	11	7

<u>FOOD GROUP VI</u>

BEANS	Amt	Cal	Prot/g	Carb/g	Fat/g
Black beans, boiled	8 oz	299	20	54	1
Kidney beans, boiled	8 oz	288	20	52	1
Lima beans, boiled	8 oz	261	18	47	1
Navy beans, boiled	8 oz	322	20	60	2
Split peas, boiled	8 oz	267	19	48	1
Tofu, plain	4 oz	75	8	2	5

GLUTEN-FREE STARCHES	Amt	Cal	Prot/g	Carb/g	Fat/g
Brown rice, cooked	8 oz	251	6	52	2
Corn tortilla	1 ea	67	2	14	1
Potato, baked	7 oz	220	5	32	3
Popcorn, air-popped/plain	2 oz	216	7	44	3
Sweet potato, baked	4 oz	60	1	14	3
Waffle, gluten-free/plain	1 ea	218	5	26	10
Winter squash, baked	8 oz	88	2	20	2

STARCHES WITH GLUTEN	Amt	Cal	Prot/g	Carb/g	Fat/g
Bagel, whole wheat plain	1 ea	187	7	36	1
Bread, whole wheat slice	1 ea	86	4	16	2
Corn muffin	2 oz	173	4	29	5
Lasagna pasta, cooked	4 oz	60	6	32	1
Oatmeal, plain	8 oz	133	6	23	2
Pancake, whole wheat 5"	1 ea	108	5	15	4
Pasta spirals, cooked	4 oz	160	6	32	1

Chapter 8

Variations for Rotating High-Carb and Low-Carb Meals

How to Make The Fat Burning Diet Fit YOUR Lifestyle

The Diet is Easy to Adjust

The key to success with The Fat Burning Diet is to make the diet work with YOUR lifestyle. The Fat Burning Diet is very easy to adjust so that it meets your needs. If you find the traditional way of following the diet is not ideal for you (i.e. is not compatible with your lifestyle), then simply adjust the low-carb high-carb eating patterns to fit your needs and lifestyle.

When starting the diet, it is ideal to keep the one-day low-carb/one-day high-carb pattern in place for the first 30 days or until you are comfortable with the program. Once you are comfortable with the eating plan, then you may alter the low-carb/high-carb patterns to fit YOUR lifestyle.

Calories Count

Keep in mind that calories DO count. Cutting carbs is only half the equation. You must also eat fewer calories each day to induce weight loss. Once you reach your fat loss goal, simply keep calories low enough to maintain your weight.

The Fat Burning Diet

VARIATIONS OF THE FAT BURNING DIET

NOTE: Low-carb days dictate that starches, sweets, and sweet fruits are avoided—yet carbohydrates (in moderation) are still consumed in the form of non-starchy vegetables, dairy products, and one or two servings of low-carb fruit.

1. "Two Low"
In one day you consume two low-carb meals and one high-carb meal.
Application: Daily low-carb twist for low-to-moderately active individuals.

2. "Two High"
In one day you consume two high-carb meals and one low-carb meal.
Application: Daily higher-carb twist for active individuals.

3. "Maxi-Burn"
Two low-carb days followed by one high-carb day.
Application: Provides maximum fat burning when preparing for a bodybuilding contest, transformation contest, or for short periods to lower body fat rapidly.

4. "One-Meal Deal"
One low-carb meal followed by one high-carb meal—then repeat cycle.
Application: Meal-to-meal variation of the traditional diet plan.

5. "Glycogen Expander I"
One low-carb day followed by three very high-carb days; then repeat cycle.
Application: Glycogen expander for runners, triathletes, and all endurance athletes.

6. "The Weight Gainer"
Three high-calorie high-carb days followed by one low-to-moderate calorie low-carb day; then repeat cycle.
Application: For gaining weight (eating high-calorie meals for gaining muscle).

7. "Glycogen Expander II"
Two low-carb days followed by two high-carb days.
Application: To help expand glycogen storage capacity in moderately active individuals.

8. "Glycogen Expander III"
Four low-carb days followed by three high-carb days to replenish glycogen.
Application: Another technique to help expand glycogen storage capacity in moderately active individuals. This technique is radical and will drive your glycogen levels extremely low. This is not advised for very active individuals or athletes.

9. "The Banquet Buster"
Eat two low-calorie low-carb meals prior to your event to deplete glycogen and prepare your body for a larger calorie and carbohydrate intake. Once you have prepared for the event, you may enjoy the food without guilt!
Application: This is a special technique to prepare for a special occasion, banquet, dinner, or celebration that will place you in front of a lot of high-calorie high-carb foods.

10. "The Alkaline Cleanse"
Eat only non-starchy vegetables, starchy vegetables, fresh vegetable juice, and fresh fruits for one full day.
Application: To alkalize and help cleanse the body of toxins. Can be used one to four times a month with good results.

11. "Two Meals a Day—Traditional"
Drink water (or perhaps eat one or two pieces/servings of fresh fruit) until noon. Follow the traditional one-day low-carb and one-day high-carb eating pattern; then repeat cycle. Because calo-

ries are low in the morning, be sure to consume enough calories in your two main meals to keep your metabolism from slowing down.

Application: For those who don't have time—or don't desire—to have breakfast.

12. "Two Meals a Day—Split"

Drink water (or perhaps eat one or two pieces/servings of fresh fruit) until noon. Then eat a low-carb lunch and a high-carb dinner *or* a high-carb lunch and a low-carb dinner. Because calories are low in the morning, be sure to consume enough calories in your two main meals to keep your metabolism from slowing down.

Application: For those who don't have time—or don't desire—to have breakfast.

Jesus said, "I am the vine, and you
are the branches."
—John 15:5 CEV

Chapter 9
Jay's 10 Laws of Digestion

"I know God will not give me anything I can't
handle. I just wish He didn't trust me so much."
—Mother Teresa

Eating foods that digest well together is very important to good
health and permanent weight control. If the foods you consume
do not digest completely, then undigested food particles can be
present in your system, and your body won't know what to do
with them.

The carbohydrate portion of your food is designed to break
down into glucose and be used for energy or stored for later
use. Protein is designed to break down into its fundamental
amino acids so your body can use them as building blocks for
hair, skin, muscle, et cetera. Fat is designed to be broken down
and used as an energy source to help lubricate your system or
to be stored as fat for future energy needs.

Should any of the protein, fat, or carbohydrate mentioned above
fail to be broken down and utilized properly by your body, then
undigested food particles can create allergies and allergy-like
symptoms—such as headaches, sneezing, mucus, post nasal
drip, dry throat, arthritis, swollen joints, skin rashes, and itchy
eyes. Undigested nutrients and unabsorbed food particles can
also be stored or suspended in the body in the form of moles,
mucous, tabs, warts, cysts, calcium deposits, and bone spurs.

On the following two pages, I have listed my *10 Laws of
Digestion and Food Combining* so you can get the most from
the foods you consume.

Jay's 10 Laws of Digestion
and Food Combining

1. FEED the lactobacteria in your colon with 1-2 tablespoons of lactose-rich sweet dairy whey two to five days a week. On high-carb days, whole food starches—such as potatoes, yams, sweet potatoes, winter squash, and brown rice—will also help feed the lactobacteria in your colon.

2. FOR BEST DIGESTION, meals that are high in carbohydrate should be low in protein, and meals that are high in protein should be low in carbs.

3. EAT MELONS alone as the first meal of the day. Eating melons with other foods, including other fruits, can lead to gas and bloating.

4. FRUIT should not exceed more than one piece, or serving, at any meal. Sweet fruits should be eaten with high-carb meals, and low-to-medium-carb fruits should be eaten with low-carb meals. If an abundance of fruit is desired, consume it alone and at breakfast only.

5. AVOID STARCHES on low-carb days to maximize digestion. On high-carb days, consume starches. It's that simple.

6. ALLOW 4-6 HOURS to pass between meals to ensure complete digestion. Eating sooner can easily interrupt the digestion of the previous meal and lead to gas, bloating, poor digestion, and poor elimination.

7. SNACKS should be avoided unless you are extremely active and need the extra calories to maintain your weight and performance. It is still ideal to allow at least four hours to pass between meals or snacks to ensure good digestion.

8. WHEAT and all grains (except millet and brown rice) should be avoided unless you pass *Jay's Wheat and Gluten Test* (See pages 56-57). If you pass the test and do consume whole wheat and other whole grains, they should only be consumed on high-carb days.

9. MILK and dairy products should be nonfat or low-fat and lactose-free (lactose converted) if you are sensitive to lactose. If milk does not digest well for you, then avoid it and focus on nonfat or low-fat plain yogurt for your dairy intake.

10. 12 HOURS should pass between the last meal of the day and the first meal of the following day. This will ensure that you have completely digested and assimilated the food from the previous day. It will also ensure that you have timely and well-formed bowel movements.

"Think positive thoughts, and experience positive results. Think negative thoughts, and experience negative results. Be thought-free, and experience reality."
—The Author

Chapter 10

Feeding the Family Fat Burning Foods

"Last week our teenage son discovered
something amazing. The volume knob
also turns to the left."
—The Author

While it is often easy for one family member to change his or
her diet, expecting the rest of the family to follow suit is another matter entirely. Perhaps one of the biggest challenges concerning diet change is getting kids to eat healthy foods that are
low in sugar, refined grains, and refined carbohydrate.

Growing children can usually eat more natural carbohydrate
than adults and get away with it, meaning that children typically are active enough to burn most of the excess carbohydrate in
their diet. An optimum diet for children limits or restricts all
refined sugar and carbohydrate and leans heavily towards a balanced diet of complete proteins, essential fats and oils, non-
starchy vegetables, fruits, nuts, seeds, whole grains, and
starchy vegetables.

How Can You Get *Your* Children to Eat Correctly?

Just do your best, pray for your children, and pray for support in
your efforts. The sooner you introduce your children to whole
foods, the better. Restricting all sugar, sweets, candy, and
excess carbohydrate can, at first, appear to be an impossible
feat. Peer pressure combined with TV ads and an early-devel-
oped sweet tooth will almost always keep your child's hand in
the cookie jar.

Raising a Healthy Child Is Fun!

Never Sick His First Five Years!

Our son Angelo was born (an underwater birth) at our home in San Diego. He has been raised with love, attention, and plenty of organically grown whole foods. Being breast-fed from day one and receiving nothing but raw organically grown fruits and vegetables and breast milk his first year, our son got off to a very healthy start. In fact, Angelo was NOT SICK (with the exception of a runny nose one day when he was teething) the first FIVE years of his life. I am telling you this not to brag about our son or our accomplishments as parents; I am telling you this so you will know what *is* possible—even in America, the junk-food jungle.

Fun, Fun, Fun with Our Son!

Imagine, as parents, what it was like having a child who never got sick the first five years of his life. NO colds, sore throats, chest congestion, measles, mumps, chicken pox, fevers, vomiting, foul-smelling bowel movements, ear infections, foul-smelling diapers, doctor bills, antibiotics, medicine—and NO sleepless nights! Just fun, fun, fun with our son! How did this happen? It wasn't a coincidence. First and foremost, Rosemary and I prayed together every night for nutritional guidance. Then we simply listened to the Lord.

Here is the Breakdown of Our Nutrition Plan for Angelo:

1. He was breast-fed for three years—then intermittently the fourth and fifth year. We let HIM wean himself when HE was ready, not when we thought it convenient to stop.

2. He consumed only breast milk and raw organic fruits and vegetables until he was 13 months old. His favorite meal was fresh applesauce made in a blender. He would consume 2-4 cored and peeled apples at one sitting and loved every bite.

3. He was fed NO—and I mean NO—cereals or starches until he was over 12 months old. We tried feeding him oatmeal as a test when he was 10 months old, but after bite number two he quickly vomited it to get it out of his system. In general, children do not secrete adequate enzymes to break down starches until they are past one year of age. This could easily explain why many children vomit and have upset stomachs, gas, foul-smelling bowel movements, nasal congestion, earaches, sore throats, and colds in their early years.

4. From 13-18 months, we gradually introduced organic meat, protein drinks (made only with a low-carb high-quality protein powder), vegetables, potatoes, sweet potatoes, yams, and squash.

5. Grains were limited to only brown rice, and it was only eaten occasionally. For starches, Angelo consumed potatoes, yams, sweet potatoes, and winter squash.

6. Avocados, olive oil, flax seed oil, raw nuts, and raw seeds were sources of healthy fat in his diet.

7. Sugar was only consumed a handful of times the first five years of his life—usually at a birthday party—and we limited the amount and frequency.

8. NO pizza, refined white flour, pasta, white bread, or junk food was consumed. One month after Angelo's first birthday, his diet consisted of the basic foods in The Fat Burning Diet—i.e, vegetables, lean protein, fresh fruit, starchy vegetables, avocados, healthy fats, brown rice, and breast milk, as he desired.

9. Ice cream, cake, soda, pasteurized fruit juice, and sweets were completely avoided.

10. Fresh vegetable juices (not canned or bottled) were also included in his diet several times a week.

11. Desiccated liver tablets were introduced into his diet at about 18-20 months of age. Angelo would chew three tablets daily with meals. (The tablets can also be crushed in a pill crusher and sprinkled over vegetables or in a protein drink.) As a teen now, he currently consumes 3-5 desiccated liver tablets 3-4 days a week.

12. At 12 months, we introduced an egg white protein powder (and later a whey protein) into his diet. We made his drinks with water, fresh fruit, and flax seed oil—or unsalted nut butters.

We Postponed the Inevitable

After Angelo turned five years old, it was harder for us to monitor his every bite. And soon he began to indulge in less than wholesome foods at parties and friends' homes. Angelo caught his first cold soon after his fifth birthday due to his new dietary flexibility.

As Angelo entered his teens, he learned that his diet kept him healthy and free from illness. Now, if he eats junk food, sugar, or too much fat, he realizes it can (and oftentimes does) make him sick. He knows from personal experience WHY he gets sick, and he knows that he can avoid illness and the misery it brings just by eating healthy foods. Sometimes pain is our best teacher and getting sick can be painful enough to teach us to eat better.

Angelo is also given sweet dairy whey mixed in yogurt two to three mornings a week for breakfast to help feed the friendly bacteria in his colon, which, in turn, boosts his immune system and keeps him healthy (even when he does deviate from his diet). Sweet dairy whey can be introduced into a child's diet after one year of age—or soon after he or she is weaned. While a child is breastfeeding, sweet dairy whey is not needed.

I firmly believe in teaching our children HOW to eat and then allowing them to experience the pain of ill health if they choose to ignore the guidance of their parents. I also believe in teaching our children by EXAMPLE, not words. What you eat as a parent will have a greater impact on your children than what you try to TELL them. It is hard to tell your child that sodas, pizza, sweets, ice cream, and junk food are bad for them if you eat those foods on a regular basis.

Refined Carbohydrates Are Everywhere!

From soda pop to pizza, refined carbohydrate temptations are everywhere. Right in your own home is the first place to begin weeding out the *junk*. Go through your cabinets and perform a serious refined carbohydrate cleanse. Get rid of all the ooey, gooey products that are going to give you and your family an insulin rush. Next, replace all the junk with real foods. Begin developing meals that are centered around protein and vegetables. Stop serving pasta and macaroni and cheese as main courses, and focus on salads, steamed vegetables, potatoes, yams, squash, fruit, nuts, and lean protein.

You Deserve the Absolute Best!

Buy organically grown foods to help stop pollution and to ensure that what you serve your family is not chemically poisoned. And this goes for meats, too! Buy hormone-free meats that come from animals fed natural foods and raised under humane and healthy conditions. Ask the manager of your local supermarket to carry the above types of clean, pure foods, or simply make a choice to do all your shopping at health food stores that carry only natural foods.

For desserts, utilize many of the natural treats you'll find in the dessert section of Chapter 19. Choose vegetables, fruit, potatoes, yams, sweet potatoes, brown rice, and squash as your child's natural carbohydrate sources. Try to limit *refined starchy* foods—such as white bread, pasta, and white rice—but there is no need to go overboard. Whole grains and starchy vegetables are just fine for active children and will do no harm (unless they are allergic to the food itself, which is especially true if body temperatures are low and thyroid output is weak).

Make Dietary Transition Fun

Do your best to raise your children on whole unrefined foods, but don't force the action. Let it flow, especially if radical dietary changes are necessary. Forcing your children to change against their will can often create attitudes of resentment toward wholesome foods that may lead down the road to complete rebellion. Keep it light, *set a good example*, and make dietary transition a fun and memorable experience for the entire family.

> "All things whatsoever you shall ask in prayer, believing, you shall receive."
> —Matthew 21:22

Chapter 11

Dining Out Made Easy

"Make every day a holiday and every
meal a fat burning banquet!"
—The Author

There you sit facing a menu that is loaded with every no-no on the planet. You are salivating as the waiter asks, "What will you have?" You are tempted to blurt out, "One of each," but you look on your right shoulder and see me sitting there watching you. So instead of losing control, you quickly reply, "It's a low-carb day, so I'll have the large salad, grilled salmon, and Italian dressing on the side. And please don't bring any bread to the table." The waiter replies, "Healthy choice." You did it!

Millions of individuals blow their diet as soon as they leave their home and enter uncharted waters—usually their favorite restaurant. On my Fat Burning Diet, it's fun and easy to dine out.

Because of my busy schedule, I eat about half my meals away from home. Due to my hectic schedule that forces me to dine out often, I have become an expert at ordering according to The Fat Burning Diet principles.

Below are options you can exercise when you visit your favorite dining establishment:

NOTE: It is ideal to request ice water with your meal and a slice or two of lemon or lime. Squeeze the lemon or lime into the water, and add granulated stevia powder to the mixture to give it a sweet taste without the use of sugar or additional carbohydrate. This quick limeade/lemonade will give you a healthy dose of alkaline minerals, Vitamin C, and bioflavonoids. It will also save you money. (The average price of a beverage at a restaurant is approximately $1.50. If you purchased one beverage every day, you would spend $547.50 in one year.)

BREAKFAST DINERS

Low-carb days:
- Eggs
- An omelet
- Tomatoes
- Cottage cheese
- Lean sausage
- Canadian bacon
- Hamburger patty
- Lean steak
- Slices of turkey breast
- A chicken breast
- Strawberries, a grapefruit, or an orange

High-carb days:
- Eggs
- Lean meat
- Hash browns (request they are cooked with very little oil)
- Skillet potatoes
- Rice cereal
- Corn tortillas
- Avocado slices
- A banana

NOTE: Waffles, pancakes, oatmeal, toast, bagels, and French toast are usually made with wheat and contain gluten. If you are absolutely certain that wheat and gluten are not problems for you, then you may occasionally order these foods that contain wheat. But don't make a habit of it. The wheat used is almost always refined bleached white flour, containing almost no fiber or nutrition. When consuming these foods, I highly advise taking a full-spectrum digestive enzyme to help break down the food properly.

MEXICAN

Low-carb days:
- Grilled chicken, fish, or beef
- Large salad
- Salsa and/or dressing of choice
- Black beans or refried beans

Skip the chips.

High-carb days:
- Avocado slices
- Bean tostadas
- Beans
- Chicken, beef, or fish enchiladas
- Chicken, beef, or fish tacos
- Chips and salsa (go easy)
- Corn tortillas
- Guacamole
- Rice
- Rice and bean enchiladas
- Rice and bean tacos

NOTE: Burritos and flour tortillas are usually made with refined wheat flour that has been bleached. Certain healthy Mexican restaurants may offer sprouted tortillas or tortillas made with whole wheat. Only eat burritos and flour tortillas if you are absolutely sure that you are not allergic to wheat or sensitive to gluten.

ITALIAN

Italian restaurants are mini-wheat factories, so save these ethnic restaurants for your once-a-week FREE MEAL, if possible. That is what I do. Should you find yourself parked at an Italian restaurant table and it is not time for your FREE MEAL, then God help you. Try the following:

Low-carb days:
- Grilled chicken, fish, or beef
- Large salad
- Dressing

Skip the breadbasket. Don't even let them put it on your table!

High-carb days (FREE MEAL):
- Just about anything on the menu will do for carb-loading at your FREE MEAL. Don't make carb-loading at Italian restaurants a habit; use your digestive enzymes.

CHINESE, THAI, JAPANESE, VIETNAMESE, AND SUSHI BARS

Low-carb days:
- Vegetables
- Chicken, fish, turkey, or beef

Skip the rice and high-carb appetizers.

High-carb days:
- Vegetables (any and all)
- Brown rice (or white rice if that's all they have)
- Chicken, beef, or fish with rice dishes are excellent
- Tofu—steamed, not fried, if given choice
- Spring rolls or egg rolls (avoid if fried)

AVOID noodle dishes unless they are rice noodles. And do not indulge in the fried crispy noodles they sometimes offer as a complimentary appetizer before your meal is served.

GREEK

Low-carb days:
- Chicken, fish, turkey, or beef
- Greek salad
- Steamed vegetables
- Sliced tomatoes

High-carb days:
- Greek restaurants usually only have wheat-based products so, like Italian restaurants, it is best to eat Greek food for your once-a-week FREE MEAL. If not, take your enzymes, and don't make a habit of carb-loading in Greece. Table-dancing anyone?

INDIAN

Low-carb days:
- Vegetables
- Any and all meats
- Cream sauces

High-carb days:
- Vegetables
- Meat dishes
- Rice
- Rice crackers or bread

NOTE: Most of their breads are wheat-based, so avoid—except for those special occasions.

The Fat Burning Diet

SEAFOOD

Low-carb days:
- Salads
- Vegetables
- Fish, fish, and more fish!
- All seafood—not fried

Skip the breadbasket.

High-carb days:
- Salads
- Vegetables
- Fish and seafood, not fried
- Potatoes, squash, or sweet potatoes
- Breadbasket (best for FREE MEALS only)

Go light on the butter and fats.

STEAKHOUSE

Low-carb days:
- Salads
- Vegetables
- Steaks or any meat

High-carb days:
- Salads
- Vegetables
- Beef or meat dishes (go small and light)
- Potatoes, squash, or sweet potatoes
- Breadbasket (best for FREE MEALS only)

Go light on the butter and fats.

LUNCH DINER

Low-carb days:
- Salad
- Plain burger (no bun), lean steak, chicken, fish, or turkey
- Vegetables (no potatoes)
- Cottage cheese
- Low-carb fruit plate or an apple (if available)

High-carb days:
- Salad
- Vegetables
- Meat of choice, not fried
- Potatoes, squash, or sweet potatoes

FAST FOOD (BURGERS)

Low-carb days:
- 1-2 large burgers with or without cheese (no bun)
- Salad bar (if available)
- Tomato slices
- Cottage cheese (if available)

That's about it for burger joints.

High-carb days:
- Salad bar (if available)

There is usually nothing else worth eating.

> "There can be no happiness if the
> things we believe in are different
> than the things we do."
> —Freya Stark

Chapter 12
Jay's Way to Control Diabetes

"Nothing will ever be attempted if all
possible objections must be overcome."
—Samuel Johnson

If you are a diabetic Type 2 or Type 1, then The Fat Burning Diet
should be ideal for you. You must work with your doctor, however. Diabetes Type 1 is not reversible and is usually caused by
a genetic flaw that inhibits the natural production of insulin.
Diabetes Type 2 is often reversible because it is usually 100%
self-induced due to the over-consumption of the wrong types of
carbohydrate foods, a sedentary lifestyle, and nutrient deficiencies. Following the basic principles of The Fat Burning Diet
will do wonders for both types of this disease.

**Your goal as a diabetic is to keep your blood glucose levels
within a healthy range at all times.** If you are a **Type 1 diabetic**,
then you will be utilizing exogenous (externally derived) insulin
to manage your higher carb meals. During low-carb meals, you
may need much less insulin or none at all. It is advisable to
work closely with your doctor as you cut carbs to manage your
glucose levels.

**If you are a Type 2 diabetic, then your goal is to allow your pan-
creas to rest through low-carb eating** and then use high-carb
meals intermittently, as needed, for glycogen reloading with the
timing indicated by your glucose levels. If you are an insulin-
dependent diabetic, exogenous insulin may be needed at first
to manage your higher carb meals. Over time, your body may
once again produce proper amounts of insulin that receptor

sites may recognize, thus eliminating the need to supplement with insulin injections or tablets. Your doctor can help you with this process that must be monitored carefully.

As a diabetic, your diet should be heavily focused on lean protein and vegetables. Super-sized salads, gobs of green beans, zillions of zucchinis, buckets of broccoli, crates of cabbage, and all other low-carb raw or cooked vegetables eaten in volume are ideal. The carbs in most low-carb vegetables are generally safe and ideal for the diabetic.

The 10 Keys to Managing Blood Glucose Levels for Diabetics

(See Chapter 6 for examples of low-carb and high-carb meals.)

1. Use a blood glucose monitoring device to determine when you should consume low-carb meals and when you should consume high-carb meals.

2. Eat low-carb meals until blood sugar levels are between 80-90mg/dl. Once glucose levels are under control (which may take 1-3 days of low-carb eating), make your next three meals (eaten all in one day) high in carbohydrate, utilizing lean protein, healthy fats, low-carb vegetables, and high-carb low-glycemic alkaline vegetables—such as yams, sweet potatoes, or winter squash. The purpose of these high-complex carbohydrate alkaline meals is to reload glycogen levels quickly while not overtaxing your pancreas. (Review all low-carb and high-carb meal ideas in Chapter 6.)

3. After one day of high-complex carbohydrate consumption, return the next day to low-carb meals, and continue for 1-3 days until glucose levels are consistently below 90mg/dl. Use a glucose monitor as often as needed to track your glucose levels. If your glucose level returns to normal the day after a high-carb day, you must still consume low-carb meals for at least one full day to let your pancreas rest and lower glycogen levels. Then simply repeat your carb-depleting, carb-loading cycles as indicated by your glucose meter. If you are a Type 2 diabetic, over time you should be able to handle natural carbohydrates in higher quantities. It will take time, so be patient.

4. Avoid wheat, oatmeal, and all grains, instead focusing on starchy and non-starchy vegetables for your main source of carbohydrate.

5. Initially, fruit intake should be limited to low-carb fruits—such as lemons, limes, grapefruit, oranges, apples, tangerines, strawberries, or all other berries. Do not eat fruit at high-carb meals. Fruit should also be limited to no more than two servings a day.

6. Utilize low-fat dairy products as a healthy source of carbohydrate and protein. The sugar content of dairy products (lactose) is metabolized slowly and moderately. Lactose also helps feed the healthy lactobacteria colonies that reside in your colon.

7. Eat high-fiber foods, and avoid the use of wheat bran, oat bran, and psyllium husks or seeds. Wheat bran and oat bran can be very irritating to the intestinal tract and allergenic for those sensitive to grains. Psyllium husks are a good fiber source, yet they do tend to alkalize the colon and strip it of friendly bacteria, which could lead to a dependency on this source of fiber for regularity. For added fiber in your diet, use ground flax seeds, or you may also use stabilized rice bran. You may cook with rice bran, but flax seeds should never be heated before consumption due to the delicacy of the Omega-3 oils present in them. Golden flax seeds are the best tasting of the flax varieties.

8. Read labels carefully on all foods you consume. Especially watch out for the vast number of protein bars that are on the market. Most of them contain ingredients you should be avoiding as a diabetic. Look for bars that contain xylitol as the sweetener.

9. If you know you are allergic to any specific foods, AVOID them! Diabetics are notorious for being allergic to grains, especially refined grains. Because of food allergies, diabetics are often carbohydrate addicts. Cutting carbs, avoiding allergenic foods, getting fit, and managing your glucose levels will help end your addictions to food forever!

10. Pray daily and ask God for guidance and strength. He has always kept me on track and motivated me to do my best. He can do the same for you. All you need to do is ask.

The Fat Burning Diet

Nutritional Supplements Suggested for Diabetics and those Who are Experiencing Hypoglycemia:

200 mcg chromium (as chromium picolinate, chromium citrate, or chromium polynicotinate)—taken 3 times daily.

(4) 1500-mg desiccated liver tablets—taken with a meal once a day.

250-300 mg Vitamin C from acerola berry powder—taken 3 times daily. Vitamin C is a main constituent of collagen and can help diabetics avoid the vascular deterioration that can occur when glucose levels remain too high for too long.

500-1000 mg of free-form L-Lysine—taken 3 times daily. L-Lysine is an essential amino acid that plays a major role in the formation of collagen, keeps your artery walls strong, and can boost your immune system.

4-6 tbs golden flax seeds (finely ground)—taken daily with meals. Mix with yogurt, protein drinks, or other foods.

1 tbs flax seed oil (great in a protein drink)—taken daily to supply your body with Omega-3 essential fatty acids. Omega-3 oils are especially good for keeping your nerves healthy. With peripheral neuropathy being prevalent in approximately 50% of those afflicted with blood sugar disorders, consuming essential fatty acids is critical for maintaining a healthy nervous system.

Chapter 13
Say Good-bye to Constipation, Gas, Diarrhea, and Yeast Infections

"For fast-acting relief,
try slowing down."
—Lily Tomlin

I know first-hand how uncomfortable it is to have problems with your colon. Gas, bloating, diarrhea, and constipation were very common to me throughout high school, college, and for several years thereafter until I made specific changes in my diet and lifestyle.

When I was growing up, I recall having normal bowel movements until I got into high school. By *normal bowel movements*, I mean they were well formed, left my body quickly, and didn't have an offensive odor. As I recall, all the years before high school, I didn't have any trouble with gas or bloating. But all that changed in high school.

When I turned 15, I wanted to get a job so I could save money for a car and an education. Shortly thereafter, I applied for a job at a local pizza restaurant and was hired. My first official job provided me a whopping $1.00 an hour. The year was 1968—gas prices fluctuated between 35 and 39 cents a gallon, and a movie ticket cost approximately $1.35—so I figured I could survive making one green back for every 60 minutes I made pizzas.

The best part about my job was the fact that I could eat and drink as much as I wanted while I was working. I was in heaven—or so I thought!

The Fat Burning Diet

Who said ignorance is bliss? While pizza became a daily staple for me, it is actually not considered to be a *whole food* (foods that are naturally high in fiber and key nutrients that your body needs and thrives on)—mainly because the crust is comprised of white flour. White flour is a very addictive high-glycemic-rated food that can drive a person to overeat. Pizza is also extremely high in calories, fat, and carbohydrate—making it the perfect food to swell your fat cells. I didn't know it at the time, but wheat flour can literally destroy a person's colon; nor did I know that I was gluten intolerant. And wheat is loaded with *gluten* (a protein found in certain grains). So there you have it. Working every night until one, coupled with a steady diet of pizza and beer, did *nothing* to enhance my health during my high school years.

Right now you may be thinking I was perpetually sick and missed a lot of school due to my brutal schedule, but just the opposite was true. I don't recall missing a day of work or school all through high school in spite of my workload. How did I do it? To maintain my grades, my health, and my well-being required a very strong will and the periodic use of prescription antibiotics. Several times a year, when I would develop tonsillitis, I pre-scribed to a round of antibiotics that allowed me to recover quickly and never miss a day of school or a night of work.

Unfortunately, the combination of antibiotics and the gluten in the pizza dough almost completely destroyed the friendly bac-teria in my colon. Once my friendly lactobacteria was destroyed, I developed chronic bouts of gas, bloating, bad breath, yeast overgrowth (Candida), foul-smelling bowel movements, and diar-rhea. In short, life became challenging as I felt like a hot-air bal-loon and could have single-handedly (or should I say *"single-endedly"*) supported the toilet paper industry.

I recall not being able to sit through a full-length movie at the theater without feeling like my colon would explode from the gas buildup. This made dating very difficult and life, in general, difficult. But there is a *happy ending* (pun intended) to this colon caper. Because I experienced first-hand the daily misery of Candida, gas, bloating, and foul-smelling bowel movements, I was very interested in knowing WHY I had these woes. The good news for you is that because of my diligence and discoveries, YOU, too, may be able to avoid colon problems for the rest of your life.

Constipation is a looming problem in America. How do I know this? It's easy. Laxatives and stool softeners are considered to be two of the top-selling over-the-counter drugs in America. There are a lot of constipated, bloated, and gas-filled Americans out there, and one of them may be you. This is no laughing matter.

My goal with this chapter is to teach you a simple dietary secret that can keep your colon happy and your bowel movements effortless and odorless. Please hear me out.

A healthy colon is filled with two basic types of bacteria. Approximately 80% of the bacteria present in a healthy colon should be friendly bacteria (especially lactobacteria) that aid in digestion and elimination, and approximately 20% should be harmful bacteria. The 80-20 ratio is critical to good colon health. Should anything disrupt the friendly to unfriendly bacteria balance in the colon, trouble can start brewing.

Antibiotics can save lives. Unfortunately, the overuse of antibiotics can also cause illness because antibiotics not only destroy harmful bacteria in your body, but they can also destroy the friendly bacteria (lactobacteria) in your colon.

Lactobacteria (the friendly bacteria in your colon) feeds primarily on lactose, which is the sugar found in milk and sweet dairy whey. Lactobacteria can also feed on dextrin, which is the end product of *complex carbohydrate* (primarily starch) digestion. Milk is rich in lactose, so those who consume milk daily may be able to feed their lactobacteria effectively.

The Fat Burning Diet

Many adults don't drink milk. Once an adult stops drinking milk and consuming dairy products, lactobacteria can begin to slowly die off due to starvation. The longer an adult is away from milk or lactose-rich products, the lower the lactobacteria count can get—until that same person may no longer tolerate milk or dairy products. Lactobacteria colonies need to be heavily populated in the human colon for proper digestion to take place—especially for the proper digestion of dairy products. Millions of lactose-intolerant individuals in the world could be an indicator that humans are no longer feeding their lactobacteria colonies.

Sweet Dairy Whey to the Rescue!

Sweet dairy whey, different from whey protein, is very rich in lactose and, in my opinion, is the ideal food for lactobacteria. Sweet dairy whey is the liquid that rises to the top during the process of making cheese and cottage cheese. Sweet dairy whey is then spray dried at cold temperatures to form a dry powder. Sweet dairy whey is low in protein and high in *lactose* (milk sugar). Lactose is the primary food for the lactobacteria in your colon, making sweet dairy whey an ideal supplement for feeding the friendly bacteria in your colon.

How to Feed the Lactobacteria in Your Colon:

Jay's Power Pudding
At one meal each day, do the following:
In a medium-size bowl place—
- 16 oz nonfat plain yogurt (do not use sweetened yogurt)
- 2 tbs sweet dairy whey
- 2-4 tbs golden flax seeds—ground fine
- 1 tsp granulated stevia powder

Mix these ingredients together, and enjoy this tasty dish.

On high-carb days, for variety, you may also wish to add to Jay's Power Pudding (see page 138) the following ingredients:
- 1 small banana—cut into bite-size pieces
- 2 tbs dried sweet potato cereal (yam nuggets)

On low-carb mornings, for variety, you may also wish to add to Jay's Power Pudding the following ingredients:
- 2 tbs whey protein (vanilla flavor)
- 6 ripe strawberries

Jay's Power Pudding should be consumed once a day for approximately 60 days—until bowel movements are well formed, nearly odorless, and easy to pass. For maintenance thereafter, Jay's Power Pudding can be taken 3-4 times a week to maintain a high population of lactobacteria. Sweet dairy whey can also be taken in plain water or in a protein drink.

VERY IMPORTANT NOTE ON LACTOSE INTOLERANCE:
If you are lactose intolerant, have not consumed milk for several months (or longer), or are experiencing gas, bloating, and poor bowel movements when you consume dairy products—then it is highly advisable to take a *lactase enzyme* (an enzyme that aids in the breaking down of lactose). Usually one or two capsules of a high-quality lactase enzyme is all that is needed to break down the lactose that is found in two tablespoons of sweet dairy whey.

Carb-Loading Days Can Help Feed Lactobacteria

On high-carb days, you will be consuming yams, sweet potatoes, winter squash, brown rice, and potatoes—all of which can break down to dextrin and become a secondary food for the lactobacteria population in your colon. If you are not wheat- and gluten-sensitive, you may also consume *some* whole grains—preferably those starches that are derived from vegetable sources instead of grains. Additionally, on low-carb days, harm-

139

ful bacteria—i.e., certain types of yeast—will be starved because their primary food is sugar. Yeast organisms in your colon prefer to have little competition with lactobacteria. By consuming sweets, fruit juice, desserts, ice cream, sugar, fructose, corn syrup, white flour, white bread, white pasta—any foods that convert to glucose very rapidly—you may be feeding the yeast and harmful bacteria in your colon. Those guys LOVE sweets, and part of your sweet tooth could be attributed to the yeast in your body that causes you to crave high-carb foods.

Your Colon Loves Fresh Sauerkraut!

Fresh raw sauerkraut is teeming with lactobacteria that can greatly enhance the health of your colon and ensure that bowel movements are effortless and odorless. Sauerkraut is made by naturally fermenting sliced cabbage. Sauerkraut must be raw (not pasteurized) to preserve the lactobacterial activity created during the natural fermentation process. Lactobacteria are easily destroyed by the heat during pasteurization. Raw sauerkraut is available at most health foods stores, or you may make your own. (See Homemade Sauerkraut recipe on page 211.)

In Summary

To ensure that your colon is healthy and happy, it is very important to regularly consume sweet dairy whey to help feed your friendly lactobacteria. It is also important to consume low-carb meals periodically, as suggested in this book, to help starve the yeast and unfriendly bacteria. You must also consume starches from vegetable sources to provide fiber and secondary food for the lactobacteria in your colon. And, lastly, you must avoid refined sugars, sweets, junk food, and simple sugars that can directly feed the unfriendly bacteria and yeast organisms in your colon.

Chapter 14

The Cholesterol Myth and the REAL Cause of Heart Disease

"It is better to learn
late, than never."
—Publilius Syrus

We are at war! Pick up any newspaper, magazine, or health publication, and it becomes obvious we are fighting a silent battle against CHOLESTEROL. Because cholesterol deposits itself in the arteries of heart attack victims, it has been assumed that cholesterol and the majority of fats are not healthy and should be avoided like the plague.

We have low-cholesterol cookbooks, many of our packaged foods contain no fat, and the most popular buzzword is *fat-free!* **In all this no-fat/low-fat/cholesterolphobia commotion, has anyone stopped to take a look at how important cholesterol is to our health and well-being?**

If you don't believe that diet and health are two controversial subjects, then you must be new to the field of nutrition. One study will offer specific, conclusive findings that become "dietary fact"—then two years later, another study will disprove this fact. I don't consider cholesterol to be any different. Look at how inconsistent the authorities have been on their judgment concerning eggs. One year they condemn eggs and give them a life sentence; the next, they are letting eggs out of prison and confessing they jumped to conclusions.

In fact, a recent news release stated that a panel of leading medical experts has seriously questioned the role of cholesterol in heart disease. These medical authorities feel that total restriction from eating meat and dairy products is unwarranted. It seems they realize that even though specific dietary habits can alter the level of blood cholesterol, heart disease may be linked to other factors. This panel of medical experts now believes that rather than focusing exclusively on cholesterol, a more balanced view of the connection between diet and cardiac disease should be adopted.

Cholesterol Is Vital to Your Health

Your body produces cholesterol because it is vital to your health and well-being. Even if you avoid cholesterol entirely, your body will work overtime to produce your daily needs. And no matter how much cholesterol you consume daily, your body will still only absorb approximately 300-500 milligrams, with the remainder of your cholesterol needs being produced by your liver. In fact, through very sophisticated clinical studies, it has been determined that 60-70% of all blood cholesterol is produced by the liver and not by our cholesterol-rich foods.

Cholesterol is vitally important to every cell of the body. One of cholesterol's major roles is being the substance that your body uses in the production of steroid hormones—including testosterone, estrogen, progesterone, cortisone, and aldosterone. Your skin contains large concentrations of cholesterol, and this is where your body converts it to Vitamin D in the presence of direct sunlight. Cholesterol seals off damaged tissues and arterial walls and is also needed to protect the cells of your body from being damaged by radiation, toxins, and other harmful substances. Are you beginning to understand how important cholesterol is for your body?

So how did such a wonderful and vitally important substance like cholesterol get such a bad rap? Its name has graced tabloids from here to China. I believe science was looking for something to blame as the cause for heart disease.

Cholesterol, being found deposited in the arteries of many heart attack victims, seemed like a good place to point the finger. Cholesterol just happened to be at the scene of the crime, but in America you are innocent until proven guilty. In my opinion, the combination of sugar, refined carbohydrates, excess carbohydrate consumption, processed foods, refined fats, junk food, and lack of exercise is the real culprit. Why wouldn't scientists believe that this "potpourri of goodies" could do some real damage to the heart?

As pointed out by world-famous physician Dr. Cass Igram—in his extremely popular book, *Eat Right to Live Long* (Literary Visions Publishing, Inc., 1994)—Too low of a cholesterol level is as dangerous as a cholesterol level that is too high. He then lists what he feels are the six causes of high cholesterol.

The Six Causes of High Cholesterol:

1. Excess dietary sugar
2. Excess dietary starch
3. Excess hydrogenated processed fats
4. Liver dysfunction
5. Amino acid (protein) deficiency
6. Essential fatty acid (fat) deficiency

Without Cholesterol You Would Die!

All natural foods that contain cholesterol are loaded with lecithin and other fatty acid mobilizing nutrients that keep cholesterol moving within the body so that it is able to accomplish its many vital functions. Without cholesterol, you would die! If cholesterol is at fault and the "root cause" of heart disease, why in the world would your body be producing it in such large quantities each and every day of your life?

I feel that specific vitamins and essential minerals are lacking in the diet of someone who consumes processed foods, which then causes cholesterol to behave in a gooey, binding manner. And because of serious nutritional deficiencies—especially copper, selenium, calcium, and Vitamin C—arteries and blood vessels weaken to the point of bulging and/or bursting as the cholesterol sludge pushes its way through the bloodstream. This nutritional deficiency-induced problem is then recognized as cardiovascular disease, a heart attack, and/or a stroke.

HDLs and LDLs Are Both "Good Guys"

I'm also opposed to this cholesterol-labeling idea which states that *HDL* (high-density lipoproteins) are the "good guys" and *LDL* (low-density lipoproteins) are the "bad guys." This good guy/bad guy concept originated because your liver manufactures two carrier proteins for cholesterol. LDLs carry the cholesterol out to the tissues where it can perform its magic, while HDLs carry the cholesterol back to the liver where it is then manufactured into bile salts and prepared for excretion. LDL, distributor to the tissues, is often thought to be the slow builder of arterial occlusions and blamed for placing cholesterol in the arteries.

On the other hand, HDL—by retrieving cholesterol and returning it back to the liver, which helps prevent a buildup in the arteries—has been labeled a "good guy." The truth is HDL and LDL are absolutely necessary in the cholesterol distribution process. If labels must be applied, I see them both wearing white hats, posing as good guys who are doing their part to maintain perfect harmony within the body. Balance is the key.

The Real Cause of Heart Disease

Matthias Rath, M.D. discovered the link between Vitamin C deficiency and heart disease. In 1990, he was appointed by Dr. Pauling as the first director of cardiovascular research at the prestigious Linus Pauling Institute (then located in California).

Dr. Rath's research reveals that atherosclerosis and cardiovascular disease occur exactly for the same reason that early clinical scurvy does—a deficiency of Vitamin C in the cells comprising the arterial wall. According to Dr. Rath's research, humans, unlike animals, develop heart disease because their bodies cannot produce Vitamin C. As a consequence of Vitamin C deficiency, millions of tiny cracks and lesions develop in the arterial walls. Subsequently, cholesterol, lipoproteins, and other blood risk factors enter the damaged artery or arteriole walls to repair these lesions.

The Death Sentence

Over time, LDL cholesterol deposits a buildup inside the arterial wall, creating a blockage that can, over time, lead to a heart attack (if the buildup is near the heart) and a stroke (if the blockage or hemorrhage is in or near the brain).

Cholesterol Myth Put to Rest

Most diets are low in fruits and vegetables and low in Vitamin C, which can lead to a Vitamin C deficiency. This, in time, can cause the slow buildup of cholesterol deposits in the arterial walls—which can directly lead to heart disease. In other words, cholesterol is actually the good guy that is doing his job to stop arteries from leaking.

Supplements that Can Save Millions of Lives

In my opinion, and according to Dr. Rath's research, limiting or controlling cholesterol is not the total answer to preventing heart disease. The better answer to preventing (and perhaps reversing) heart disease is to ingest Vitamin C daily along with the amino acid L-lysine, to ensure that your connective tissues are strong and arteries are not leaking.

I Personally Recommend the Following Supplements to Help Prevent Heart Disease and Atherosclerosis:

- 300 mg Vitamin C (from acerola berry powder)—taken 3 times daily with meals.

- 500-1000 mg L-Lysine (free-form))—taken 3 times daily with meals.

For more information on Dr. Matthias Rath's research, visit his website at www.dr-rath-research.org. Dr. Rath is involved in groundbreaking research on the control of cancer and other deadly diseases.

"God delays, but doesn't forget."
—Spanish proverb

Chapter 15
Jay's Way to Get Fit Fast

"If you don't scale the mountain,
you can't view the plain."
—Chinese saying

Americans have been taught to believe that the best way to burn fat and keep body fat levels low is to exercise. Every year, especially in January, millions of individuals across the nation join fitness clubs, buy fitness gadgets, and embark on exercise routines in high hopes of dropping extra pounds they accumulated the previous year. And every year millions of Americans quit the gym, let their new fitness gadgets gather dust, or stop following their workout program because they fail to lose weight the first 30-60 days.

FASCINATING FACT:
Exercise is a poor way to burn fat and lose weight. Eating is your best means of maintaining your proper weight.

Yes, exercise can be a fat burning activity. But don't plan on losing a lot of weight by exercising. A 110-pound woman running at a speed of 6.7 mph for 30 minutes will burn approximately 291 calories. A 200-pound man running at a speed of 6.7 mph for 30 minutes will only burn approximately 528 calories. But it takes only five minutes or less to ingest 300-600 calories by eating a bowl of ice cream or drinking a large sugar-sweetened soft drink. In other words, in five minutes or less, you can offset a half-hour of running. Imagine what you could "undo" in ten minutes of eating! My point? Eating, not exercising, is your best means of maintaining your proper weight.

Please don't misinterpret what I am saying: I am not discounting the importance of exercise. Rather, I am putting exercise in its proper perspective.

You Need Regular Exercise to:

1. —strengthen your heart, lungs, and vascular system.
2. —lower glycogen levels, thus inhibiting the formation of body fat.
3. —strengthen the muscles of your body.
4. —strengthen your bones and keep them flexible and dense.
5. —slow down the aging process (the muscles on a fit body stay firm regardless of one's age).
6. —increase your stamina, endurance, and energy levels.
7. —boost your immune system.
8. —train your body to burn fat and carbohydrate more efficiently.
9. —increase your VO_2 max (oxygen utilization or maximum rate of oxygen flow).
10. —be healthy and happy!

The Absolute Best Exercise for YOU!

Having owned two fitness clubs, having been involved in body-building since 1975, having been a successful personal trainer for over 10 years, and having worked with over a thousand individuals in my professional career, I can say that the best exercise is the one that you stick with your entire life. This may sound like a sweeping statement, but it is true. **Whatever form of exercise you choose to do to get fit and maintain your shape must be easy enough and enjoyable enough to do from now until the day you die—hopefully, well past the age of 120.**

Get Fit Jay's Way

Barring any physical restrictions—walking, jogging, and running are, in my opinion, the three best forms of exercise to perform. Why? Because all you have to do is stand up and start walking, jogging, or running.

NOTE: This is not to say that I don't consider other forms of exercise to be effective. They are. In fact, I love to surf. Not everyone lives near the beach, however, and owns a surfboard, so that form of exercise is impractical for the masses.

That is the great thing about walking, jogging, and running. You can walk or run any time of the year. It takes five minutes to put your shoes and shorts on, five minutes to s-t-r-e-t-c-h, and you're off and running—wherever that happens to be, including a work trip or vacation.

The Minimum Requirement to Get Fit

According to many fitness experts, the minimum requirement of activity to get fit is 12 minutes of vigorous exercise, 3 days a week—at a level that elevates your heart rate to 70-85% of your maximum heart rate.

> **HOW TO MANUALLY DETERMINE YOUR HEART RATE:**
> - Take your pulse for 15 seconds.
> - Multiply by 4.

For ease and accuracy of tracking your heart rate during exercise, I recommend you buy a heart-rate monitor and *use it every time you work out.* I have been exercising regularly for nearly thirty years, and, with the exception of surfing and swimming, I wear a heart-rate monitor at nearly every training session to ensure I get the best possible workout.

Heart-Rate Monitors

The cost for a good heart-rate monitor is very reasonable, with a quality base model starting at approximately $60. Deluxe models can cost as much as $200 but are only necessary for highly trained athletes. The $60-$100 models are more than adequate to do the job of tracking and reporting your heart rate while you exercise.

HOW TO CALCULATE YOUR HEART RATE:

To determine your training level (70% is the low end of training; 85% is the high end), simply:
- Subtract your age from 220 (your maximum heart rate).
- Multiply the remainder by .70 (for 70%), .75 (for 75%), .80 (for 80%), and .85 (for 85%).

The answer will give you the approximate number of heartbeats per minute you should elevate your heart rate during exercise. Just strap on your heart-rate monitor, put on the heart-rate monitor watch, and start exercising. Once you reach your target heart-rate level, train at that intensity for the duration of your workout (see program below).

A Lifetime Fitness Program:
(I highly suggest you wear a heart-rate monitor.)

- **First 30 days** - Fast-walking at a speed that elevates your heart rate to 70% of your maximum heart rate for 30 minutes, 3 days a week.

- **Days 31-60** - Jogging at a speed that elevates your heart rate to 75% of your maximum heart rate for 30 minutes, 3 days a week.

- **Days 61 and beyond** - Running at a speed that elevates your heart rate to 70-85% of your maximum heart rate for 30 minutes, 3 days a week. (You can train your first session of the week at 70%, the second session at 75-80%, and the third session at 85% of your maximum heart rate. Repeat the cycle the following week.)

NOTE: After six months of training, you may wish to train for 30 minutes at session one, 45 minutes at session two, and 60 minutes at session three. Then repeat the cycle. You may also want to train every other day or for five days straight—and then take two days off and repeat the cycle.

Weight Training

To strengthen the skeletal muscles, it is also advisable to include 30 minutes of weight training, two days a week, as part of your fitness program. If you are new to fitness, it is advisable to join a quality fitness club and get professional assistance to learn the proper way to lift weights. (If you are a bodybuilder, please refer to my book, *Secrets to Successful Bodybuilding Without Steroids*, for a variety of effective training routines. The book is available on-line at www.JayRobb.com, or call toll-free 1.877.JAY.ROBB.)

NOTE: If you are currently utilizing another form of exercise that is working well for you, then by all means stick with *that* program. The walking, jogging, and running suggestions in this chapter are for those who are new to exercise or are looking for a simple, accurate, and effective way to get in shape and stay that way.

> "Go down to come up and up to come down—if a man has humbled himself, he will be exalted; but if he has exalted himself, he will be humbled."
> —Rabbi Yose

"Cut your own wood, and it will
warm you twice."
—Chinese proverb

Chapter 16
Boosting a Slow Metabolism

"When all else fails, a person often turns
to God; so why wait til the last minute?"
—The Author

Your metabolism is the sum of all the chemical reactions that occur within your body. The term "metabolic rate" is often used to describe the speed at which these chemical reactions take place. All the physical and mental processes that continually occur within your body are greatly influenced by your metabolic rate. Proper enzyme function is vitally important in the regulation of your metabolism.

While your body's fuel of choice is fat, not carbohydrate, your body's temperature of choice is 98.6 degrees Fahrenheit—no more, no less. Your body is designed to operate in a very narrow temperature range. If your temperature should increase or decrease slightly, your body will adjust to quickly return you to a natural set point, called *homeostasis*.

Enzymes are protein catalysts that control every chemical reaction that takes place in your body. Enzymes in your food are very fragile and easily destroyed by heat and cooking. Within your body, enzymes are also very sensitive to temperature. Below-normal temperatures will slow enzyme activity, and above-normal temperatures abnormally increase enzyme activity.

Enzymes are comprised of long chains of amino acids that are assembled according to the genetic code of DNA. The temper-

ature and amino acid arrangement of an enzyme primarily determines its shape. If an enzyme gets too warm, it will get loose
and lose its natural shape. Just as heat distorts the shape of
an enzyme, below-normal temperatures force an enzyme to also
lose its shape, move slowly, and become too tight for normal
function.

> "If your body temperature drops as
> little as seven tenths of a degree,
> your metabolism slows down..."

Your body operates ideally at 98.6 because that is exactly the
temperature necessary for your enzymes to function at peak
efficiency. Various enzymes in your body, however, operate best
at different temperatures, with certain enzymes being greatly
affected by the slightest temperature change. If your body temperature drops as little as seven tenths of a degree, your
metabolism slows down due to the fact that your enzymes are
cooler and functioning slower than normal. **If your body contin-
ues to operate at a cooler-than-normal temperature, then your
enzyme functions become chronically slow, and your ability to
burn fat can be greatly impaired.**

If your body temperature consistently reads between a range of
96 and 97.9 degrees Fahrenheit, then your body has possibly
gone into a conservation mode that has lowered your metabolism as a natural survival reflex. Your body is a perfect design.
If times are hard and you are faced with a lot of stress and a
food shortage, your body recognizes this as possible starvation
and quickly lowers your metabolism to conserve your energy
reserves. A person with a metabolism that slows under stress
and when food is restricted is often considered to be a "good
survivor." If your metabolism did not adjust itself and you were
faced with long-term famine, you would die sooner than some-

one who possessed a metabolism that had slowed down to survival mode.

Having a perfect metabolism that is resistant to starvation is ideal if you should ever need to survive famine. But for individuals desiring to keep their body fat low, it is imperative to not get stuck in the conservation mode—as you could remain sluggish and overweight for life. Your body should make the metabolic slowing adjustment only during times of little food and greater-than-normal stress. Once enough calories are integrated back into the diet, your metabolism should become normal and your body temperature should return to the perfect fat burning temperature—98.6 degrees Fahrenheit.

What this means is that by eating a very low-calorie diet of perhaps 600-1100 calories a day for three or more days, your metabolism may slow down. A major stress—such as childbirth, divorce, excessive exercise, a car accident, loss of a job, or the death of a family member—can also lower your temperature and enzyme function, thus reducing your body's ability to burn fat. Both starvation and stress can affect your metabolic rate by triggering your thyroid gland to hormonally manipulate your body to slow down and conserve energy.

We have received hundreds of calls from frustrated individuals, perhaps just like you, who are exercising regularly, eating a low-fat high-carbohydrate low-calorie diet and just can't seem to lose excess fat. They think they are doing everything right, yet their body fat refuses to budge. Their next step, in an attempt to lower body fat, is to cut calories further, sometimes eating NO FAT along with very high-carbohydrate foods, such as grains. In desperation, they cut calories further and begin exercising harder and longer, which is exactly the opposite of what they should be doing to start burning fat.

FASCINATING FACT:
Cutting out fat, lowering calories, severely cutting carbs, and exercising harder can easily thrust a person into metabolic slow

motion—shutting down the entire fat burning process.

The human body easily adjusts its metabolism by impairing the thyroid hormone conversion of T4 to T3. Instead of creating T3 from T4, a "stressed and starved" individual will make RT3 from much of the original T4 thyroid hormone. T3 is then not available to keep the metabolism running at normal speed, thus you immediately go into conservation mode, and your body temperature consistently remains well below 98.6 degrees Fahrenheit.

The diagram depicted on the following page illustrates the thyroid system and how it affects metabolism.

Thyroid Function and Your Metabolism

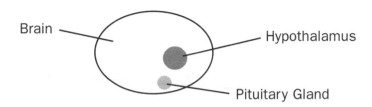

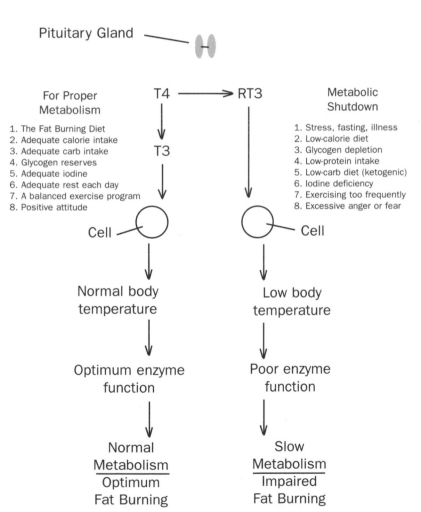

Pituitary Gland

For Proper Metabolism	T4 ⟶ RT3	Metabolic Shutdown

For Proper Metabolism

1. The Fat Burning Diet
2. Adequate calorie intake
3. Adequate carb intake
4. Glycogen reserves
5. Adequate iodine
6. Adequate rest each day
7. A balanced exercise program
8. Positive attitude

Metabolic Shutdown

1. Stress, fasting, illness
2. Low-calorie diet
3. Glycogen depletion
4. Low-protein intake
5. Low-carb diet (ketogenic)
6. Iodine deficiency
7. Exercising too frequently
8. Excessive anger or fear

T4 ⟶ RT3

T3

Cell — ◯   ◯ — Cell

Normal body temperature   Low body temperature

Optimum enzyme function   Poor enzyme function

Normal Metabolism   Slow Metabolism
Optimum Fat Burning   Impaired Fat Burning

The Fat Burning Diet

How to Easily Monitor Your Metabolic Rate

To determine if your metabolism is optimum for fat burning, simply take your temperature using an oral thermometer. To get an accurate idea of your body temperature patterns, it is best to take your temperature at various times throughout the day.

What is the Ideal Fat Burning Temperature Range?

When your metabolism is functioning optimally, you should measure approximately 97.9 degrees upon rising and then increase to 98.6 degrees within one to two hours.

FASCINATING FACT:
Most individuals begin the day a little cooler than normal. What you eat, think, and do during the day will affect your metabolism, which, in turn, will affect your body temperature.

You may employ a simple inexpensive glass oral thermometer to take your temperature, or you may find it easier to utilize the new digital styles that are now available. The digital thermometers are foolproof—easier to read and take less time to use—making it well worth the few extra dollars invested. Thermometers are available from any pharmacy. They range in price from $5 for a basic glass design up to $15 for a state-of-the-art digital model.

Stress Can Make You Chilly

If you take your temperature and you are consistently hovering around the 98.6 mark, then your metabolism is doing great. If your readings are consistently low, vacillating somewhere between 96.5 and 97.9, then it's time to stoke the fire!

As pointed out earlier, many individuals have starved themselves trying to lose weight, which actually slows their metabolism. Add the stresses of daily life and the stress of excess exercise, and your thyroid system could place you directly in survival mode, where your fat burning will stop on a dime!

Stress, by itself, can also be an underlying factor for a slow metabolism. Many individuals notice weight gains and mood swings soon after experiencing a major trauma in their life. Divorce, the death of someone close, personal injury, and loss of a job can sometimes be stressful enough to impair T4 to T3 conversion. This places you directly in the energy-conserving mode that could save your life should famine sweep the nation—or it can frustrate you if you desire to burn fat and keep your body fat at a naturally low level.

Symptoms of a Consistently Slow Metabolism

Cold hands and cold feet, and just plain being cold, is a common complaint for people with impaired metabolic rates due to improper conversion of the thyroid hormone T4 to T3. But the complaint list doesn't stop here. Allergies, asthma, itchiness, hives, unhealthy nails, acid indigestion, decreased ambition, decreased sex drive, dry skin, irregular periods, cramps, infertility, low self-esteem, slow wound healing, acne, skin infections, hemorrhoids, low-bowel motility, hypoglycemia, low blood pressure, food cravings, elevated cholesterol levels, blurred vision, carpal tunnel syndrome, psoriasis, flushing of skin (blotches) when nervous, increased bruising, ringing in the ears, canker sores, bad breath, inhibited sexual development, food intolerance, lack of coordination, profuse sweating, lack of sweating, and increased tendency to substance abuse are all common symptoms of metabolic/thyroid system malfunction.

Can't Gain Weight?

It is quite interesting to note that cold body temperatures and a slow metabolism can also prevent some individuals from gaining weight. This, I believe, is partly due to poor enzyme function, which prevents foods from being digested completely. Many times the underweight individual is also experiencing poor nutrient absorption in the small intestine due to congestion in that area of their body. A mucous-coated and congested small intestine can mean poor nutrient absorption and subsequent malnutrition, no matter how much food is eaten. Hence, the individual remains underweight even though enormous amounts of food are ingested.

What to Do If Your Body Is Running Cool:

If you have taken your temperature and discovered that you are a "cool" person, then it's time to take action and get your metabolism up to par. (You should always consult your doctor before making any serious changes in your diet and lifestyle.) The following information is a grouping of simple techniques that will help bring your metabolic rate to normal speed and get you back into fat burning mode.

1. **Eat a Fat Burning Diet** meal every 4-6 hours, three times a day. Do not miss a meal or allow yourself to become overly hungry.

2. **Begin supplementing your daily diet with** 1-2 ounces of high-quality **liquid ionic minerals.** Choose a formula that tastes good, contains 60-70 major and trace minerals, and does NOT contain artificial sweeteners. Minerals are critical to thyroid function, and a full-spectrum mineral formula is ideal for boosting the metabolism.

3. **Test yourself for iodine deficiency.** A simple home test: Swab a 3-inch by 3-inch solid square of 2% iodine tincture (the orange stuff) on your lower abdomen, and allow it to remain there for 24 hours. If the orange square disappears before the 24-hour time period, then you may need to supplement your diet with kelp and liquid iodine. Do not take high doses of a typical potassium or sodium-bound iodine supplement—as it could build up to a toxic level in your body. Use a non-toxic, water-soluble iodine to naturally replenish your iodine reserves. Kelp, dulse, and other sea vegetables are naturally rich in iodine and are a great addition to The Fat Burning Diet. Kelp is available in tablet

form for those who don't like the taste of sea vegetables.

4. **Perform a deep-breathing exercise** at least once every hour. This means you will stop what you are doing, relax, and take FIVE deep breaths—inhaling and exhaling very slowly. This deep-breathing exercise only requires about one minute to perform but can truly change your life and your metabolism by instantly reducing stress and supplying oxygen to your brain.

5. **A diet too low in carbohydrate can cause the metabolism to slow down** because the body senses it may be starving. If you are an active person, **do not carb-deplete too often or too long**, or you risk metabolic slowing, indicated by a low body temperature.

6. **Sunbathe for 15 to 30 minutes** every day, or whenever possible. Start with 5 to 10 minutes your first few times in the sun, and gradually increase your daily exposure time. Take care to never burn! The sun can naturally step up your metabolism by stimulating the thyroid gland to increase hormone production, which is the first step in maintaining a perfect metabolic rate. Experimental animals that received sunlight treatments lost weight as compared to animals given the same diet but not the sunlight treatments.

7. **Avoid cutting calories too low**. When we design calorie-specific diets for our clients, we almost never go lower than 1200 calories a day for adults. Going any lower can cause that person's metabolism to shut down and seriously impair any weight-loss efforts. I have personally witnessed individuals try to prove me wrong by cutting calories below 1000 a day only to discover that they gained weight! Once calorie intake was increased, the weight started to drop off once again. Everyone has different caloric needs, and going too far below those needs daily can cause a person to stop losing weight.

The above suggestions should return your metabolism back to a normal fat burning mode (indicated by a consistent body temperature of 98.6 degrees Fahrenheit).

If you incorporate all of these suggestions into your lifestyle and your temperature remains low, then you may have an unusually stubborn condition called Wilson's Syndrome, which may require a special T-3 hormone therapy program. (For more information on Wilson's Syndrome and to locate a physician knowledgeable in T-3 therapy, contact The Wilson's Foundation: 1.800.621.7006 / www.wilsonsthyroidsyndrome.com.)

"The best way to make your dreams come true is to wake up."
—Paul Valery

Chapter 17
Fats that Keep You Fit

"Things may come to those who wait, but
only the things left by those who hustle."
—Abraham Lincoln

- Do you crave foods high in fat?
- Do you suffer from dry skin that needs oiling on a
  daily basis?
- Have you ever followed a low-fat diet?

If you answered "yes" to *any* of the above questions, then you
need to know about the power of essential fatty acids. The word
"essential" simply means that your body cannot manufacture a
specific nutrient from another substance so that nutrient must
be consumed in the diet, or a deficiency will develop. If an
essential nutrient is not consumed in an individual's regular
diet, he or she could develop a deficiency disease—or worse,
even die from the deficiency of this nutrient.

Fat is essential to the human diet, and so is protein.
Carbohydrate is not essential. On The Fat Burning Diet, carbohydrate days are included to build up glycogen levels, provide
alkaline minerals, lighten the spirit by increasing serotonin levels, and provide short-term energy. On low-carb days, protein is
consumed to provide the amino acids needed for growth, tissue
repair, strength, muscle recovery, and stress relief. Essential
fatty acids (Omega-3 and Omega-6) and other unrefined "fat
burning fats" (as I refer to them) are consumed on low-carb and
high-carb days to provide fatty acid nutrition to the body.

FASCINATING FACT:
Eating fat is healthy. Essential fatty acids help us burn fat.

Let me repeat that. EATING FAT IS HEALTHY. But you must only consume healthy fat. Refined oils and fats are not healthy. Refined oils and fats have been altered, heated, fractionated, or processed in a way that removes the healthy components and can leave behind a fat or oil that is toxic and detrimental to your health and well-being.

Constipation, eczema-like skin eruptions, kidney problems, susceptibility to infections, sterility in males, retardation of growth, and overall weakness are but a few problems that can stem from a diet that is too low in fats (the essential fatty acids).

In his highly informative book, *Fats and Oils*, author Udo Erasmus explains that a diet high in protein but low in fat is as degenerative as a diet high in fat and low in protein. In other words, when animals were given diets deficient in protein and/or the essential fatty acids, death came quickly. In 1902, a study showed that high-carbohydrate low-protein diets result in fat deposition. High-carbohydrate high-protein diets were also found to cause an increase in fatty deposits. But when good fats were added to the same diets, less fatty deposition occurred and better food utilization and energy production took place. In other words, essential fatty acids help us burn fat, which is contrary to the average American's way of thinking.

WHERE TO GET YOUR FAT BURNING FATS
Fats are grouped as follows:

Omega-3 Family
Eicosapentaenoic Acid (EPA, 20:5w3) and Docosahexaenoic Acid (DHA, 22:6w3) is found in salmon, trout, mackerel, sardines, and other high-fat cold-water fish and marine animals. Animals that live on the land contain low amounts of EPA and DHA, *but* a high concentration of EPA and DHA can usually be found in the eyes, testes, brain, and adrenal glands of these

animals. EPA and DHA found in marine animals and land animals is the most direct way to acquire the Omega-3 essential fatty acids. Fish oil capsules can be used as an ideal source and means for attaining EPA and DHA for those who do not eat fish two to four times a week. Fish oil capsules should contain approximately 180 mg EPA and 120 mg DHA per capsule. The desired daily amount is typically 2-4 capsules.

Alpha-Linolenic Acid (LNA, 18:3w3) is found in flax seed, pumpkin seeds, walnuts, and dark green vegetables. Flax seed oil contains approximately 57% linolenic acid and is one of the richest sources of this essential fatty acid. Flax seed oil tastes great in protein drinks or can be used as a salad oil. Do not cook with flax oil. Linolenic acid is highly sensitive to heat and light, so once purchased, flax oil should be refrigerated, kept from strong light, and consumed within 60 days.

The Omega-6 Family

Linoleic Acid (LA, 18:2w6) is best found in sunflower seeds, sunflower oil, safflower oil, walnuts, walnut oil, sesame seeds, sesame oil, and flax seed oil. Sunflower seeds, sunflower oil, and safflower oil are the richest sources of this essential fatty acid.

Gamma-linolenic Acid (GLA, 18:3w6) can usually be created by the body from linoleic acid but is also found in mother's milk, borage oil, and evening primrose oil.

Arachidonic Acid (AA, 20:4w6) is found in meats and animal products.

Omega-9 Family

Oleic Acid (OA, 18:1w9) is found in olives, olive oil, almonds, almond butter, pecans, cashews, filberts (hazelnuts), and macadamia nuts.

Saturated Fat Family

Stearic Acid (SA, 18:0) is found in beef, mutton, and pork.

The Fat Burning Diet

Palmitic Acid (PA, 16:0) is found in coconuts and coconut oil. Butyric Acid (BA, 4:0) is found in butter and cream.

Keep in mind that many foods contain one dominant fat or oil, yet they also contain a mixture of other essential and non-essential fats and oils.

The Best Fats and Oils to Consume:

Fat Burning Fats are the fats and oils your body wants and needs in order to be healthy. It is important to include a variety of fats and oils in your diet for balanced nutrition. Omega-3 oils may be fantastic oils, but if you consume more of them than other oils, it can thin your blood too much and, in general, be unhealthy. Saturated fats may be the most difficult to digest and have been associated with cardiovascular disease and, in some studies, cancer. However, in reality, saturated fats are important to consume. The key is to eat a wide variety of fats and oils and to keep your fat intake moderate—ranging from 20-45% of your total calorie intake.

On low-carb days, your fat intake ratio will be higher and as much as 40-50% of your calories because carbohydrate may be as low as 10-25% of your total calories. On high-carb days, where carbohydrate may elevate to 50-70% of your total calories consumed, fat intake may drop to 15-30%, which is ideal on days you are loading carbs and glycogen. And during both days, you will be consuming a wide variety of Omega-3, Omega-6, Omega-9, and saturated fats—all derived from raw nuts, raw seeds, cold-pressed oils, lean beef, chicken, turkey, fish, golden flax seeds, flax seed oil, and fish oil capsules that are rich in EPA and DHA.

The Most Important Oils to Supplement:

Most diets are rich in a variety of fats and oils but are usually low in the Omega-3 Essential Fatty Acids. For this reason, it is important to supplement your diet with fish oil capsules and/or to consume golden flax seeds (ground fine) or flax seed oil. Fish oil is the most direct way to get Omega-3 EFAs into your system—flax seeds and flax seed oil are a close second. Both can usually be obtained from your local health food store or purchased on-line at a high-quality nutrition website.

Omega-3 Oils May Assist with:

1. High-cholesterol levels
2. High-triglyceride levels
3. Prevention of strokes and heart attacks
4. High blood pressure
5. Arthritis
6. Multiple Sclerosis
7. Psoriasis and eczema
8. Cancer prevention and treatment
9. Athletic performance
10. Dry skin

Protein Drinks Taste Delicious with Finely Ground Golden Flax Seeds and/or Flax Seed Oil

Many of my famous protein drink recipes include a high-quality egg white or whey protein mixed with freshly ground flax seeds or flax seed oil. To the best of my knowledge, I was the first health and fitness professional to advocate that athletes use flax oil at meals and in protein drinks. I have been recommending that flax oil be used in protein drinks since 1987. Most typical protein drinks are made with nonfat ingredients, which means the drink is void of essential fats and oils. Add in one tablespoon of fresh flax oil or two tablespoons of finely ground golden flax seeds to each protein drink, and you can experience the health and fitness benefits of the essential fatty acids.

NOTE: Organically grown golden flax seeds are your best choice and taste far superior to brown flax seeds. To grind flax seeds, place 3-4 tablespoons in a blender or coffee grinder, and buzz on high for 20-30 seconds—until finely ground. Store any unused flax seeds (ground or whole) in the refrigerator to preserve their freshness.

"There are no shortcuts to any place worth going."
—Beverly Sills

Chapter 18

Bodybuilding:
Bulking Up and Getting Shredded

"If you think small, you'll stay small."
—Ray Kroc

Bodybuilding is a unique sport that I personally feel is more of an art than a sport.

THE OBJECT OF BODYBUILDING:

1. To increase the size of each major muscle proportionally.

2. To lower body fat levels to a point where muscles and veins become clearly visible (termed "getting cut," "ripped," or "shredded").

The above is achieved through a regimen of training with weights, performing cardiovascular exercises, and eating a special diet that feeds the muscles and starves the fat cells. Feeding the muscles and starving the fat cells is what we will focus on in this chapter that I have divided into two parts. Part One speaks to those interested in bulking up, and Part Two speaks to those interested in getting shredded.

Part One: Bulking Up
How to pack on 20-30 solid pounds in 12-24 months.

Many bodybuilders erroneously believe they can *bulk up* (gain muscular size) while simultaneously getting *shredded* (radically lowering body fat).

The Fat Burning Diet

FASCINATING FACT:
In reality, gaining muscle while cutting calories is nearly impossible for the drug-free bodybuilder. Let me explain.

Bodybuilders who choose to use illegal steroids and other anabolic drugs to gain size and lose fat can actually gain muscle while trimming down due to the anabolic effect of the drugs they are taking. Taking drugs, such as steroids, is a dead-end street, however, that can destroy one's health and mental well-being. So taking drugs is not really an option for the serious health-conscious "natural" bodybuilder.

Q. How can I achieve success as a natural bodybuilder?

A. For the drug-free bodybuilder, the correct approach to success is to first spend 12 to 24 months on a bulking cycle followed by a 12- to 18-week cutting cycle. This unique pattern of eating and training allows bodybuilders to consume enough calories to gain all the size God intended for them to gain from lifting weights. Once maximum size is attained on the bulking phase, then most of that muscle can be maintained on the cutting phase, which can radically lower the body fat level of the bodybuilder.

Without the bulking phase, bodybuilders generally will be limited in the size they can gain because limiting calories to maintain low body fat levels is not conducive to maximum muscle growth. Once a bodybuilder packs on all the beef he or she can through high-calorie eating and serious weight training, it is relatively easy to keep that muscle through a unique cutting phase (see Part Two of this chapter).

Over the years, I have discovered that consistent low-carb eating limits muscle growth because strict low-carb diets keep insulin secretions low. Insulin is an ANABOLIC hormone that can help you build MUSCLE and FAT. Because insulin can build fat, you must control its secretion during both the bulking and cutting phase of the diet.

How the Bulking Phase Works

To gain size you must eat more food than you need to maintain your current weight. This simply means you will eat three large meals every day—eating just beyond the point you are full at each meal. Then allow your body to fully digest each meal before consuming the next meal. This will ensure that you are getting the most out of every calorie you eat.

To Gain Muscle Quickly, First Build a Strong Digestive System

To effectively gain muscular weight, it is critical that a body-builder's digestion is operating at its PEAK. If a bodybuilder is not breaking down his or her food properly, then undigested food particles may be leaking into the system and/or sliding into the small intestine and colon where they can rot and putre-fy, cause gas and discomfort, and generate poor bowel movements.

The Three Keys to Good Digestion
—and More Lean Mass:

KEY #1
The first key to good digestion is to only consume three meals a day and allow at least 4-6 hours between meals. I know this is contrary to popular opinions by many nutritionists who rec-ommend eating 5-6 small meals a day. Having experienced both ways of eating, I must recommend the more sane approach, which is to eat only three meals a day, avoiding all snacks between meals. Three meals a day allows for optimum diges-tion, which is critical for athletes and for bodybuilders. Also, if you try to consume 5-6 meals a day, you will soon find that all you are doing is shopping, preparing meals, and eating every two hours! There is more to life than shopping and eating, so

trust me on this. Eat three good meals each day, and watch yourself grow big, strong, and healthy.

KEY #2

The second key to good digestion is to AVOID: sweets, sugar, refined foods, refined fats and oils, processed meats, sucralose, aspartame, acesulfame-K, acesulfame potassium, artificial sweeteners, artificial colors, artificial flavors, fructose, white flour, white bread, white pasta, and white rice. Your body is not designed to consume artificial foods, fractionated foods, or processed foods. Your body needs whole foods, period! Whole foods are naturally high in fiber and offer key nutrients that your body needs and thrives on. To effectively avoid processed foods, you will need to read ALL labels carefully on packaged and canned foods, protein powders, protein bars, energy drinks, and energy bars.

KEY #3

To gain the size you desire, it is critical you build a powerful lactobacteria army in your colon. On the inside lining of a healthy colon resides a variety of beneficial bacteria and a variety of harmful bacteria. In a healthy colon, beneficial bacteria dominate harmful bacteria with approximately 80% of the bacteria being beneficial (including lactobacteria) and about 20% being harmful bacteria (including Candida Albicans yeast organisms). The use of antibiotics, steroids, and birth control pills, and the consumption of sugar, sweets, junk food, refined foods, bottle fruit juice, soda pop, candy, ice cream, and desserts can upset the bacteria balance in a healthy colon. Sugar and sweets feed yeast organisms and other harmful bacteria in the colon; and antibiotics, steroids, and birth control pills can destroy lactobacteria and other friendly bacteria in the colon.

To build a powerful lactobacteria army, you need to feed them daily with their favorite food, which is *lactose* (milk sugar found in sweet dairy whey and milk). One to two tablespoons of sweet dairy whey (found at your local health store) mixed in with 8-16 ounces of nonfat plain yogurt is enough food for your lactobacteria to multiply on and thrive each day. This sweet dairy whey and yogurt mixture can be consumed at any meal and can be taken up to three times a day. You will know when the sweet dairy whey is doing its job when you notice your bowel movements are perfectly formed, leave the body with little effort, and are nearly odorless. (For more information on colon health and lactobacteria feeding, see Chapter 13.)

Weight-Gainer Protein Drink—an Easy Way to Gain Size

One simple way to gain weight is to add in two or three extra protein drinks a day, consumed with meals. Below is a 350- to 450-calorie bulking phase protein drink you can consume with two to three of your daily meals to gain more size. To gain the size you desire, use the ingredients listed, *and don't make any substitutions.*

Weight-Gainer Protein Drink
In a blender, place:
- 24 oz water or nonfat milk (use lactose-free milk if you are lactose intolerant, or take a lactase enzyme)
- 4 tbs dried sweet potato cereal (or powder)
- 2 tbs whey or egg white protein powder (vanilla is best)
- 2 tbs golden flax seeds (ground fine)
- 1 tbs sweet dairy whey
- 1 tbs peanut butter, almond butter, or flax seed oil
- 1 tsp granulated stevia powder
- 3-4 ice cubes (optional)

Mix until creamy smooth, and consume with a meal.

Bulking Phase Diet Sample

The diet below is not calorie specific, so you will need to adjust the amount of food you consume to ensure it is high enough in calories to allow you to gain size and muscle mass. Nothing is more frustrating than busting your buns in the gym for months on end and gaining little to no extra mass for all your efforts. It is best to eat only three meals a day and avoid snacks to ensure you are completely digesting your foods.

NOTE: You may wish to start the first month with only one extra protein drink. Add in a second one on month two and a third on month three—consuming three drinks from that point forward. If body fat levels get too high at any time during the bulking phase, consume one day of low-carb meals every 3-5 days as needed. (For low-carb menu examples, see pages 176-178.)

High-Calorie Bulking Phase Diet Sample

BREAKFAST
- 16 oz nonfat plain yogurt mixed with 1 tbs sweet dairy whey
- 1 very large potato made into one hash brown (or two servings of hash browns) *or* 2-3 slices of gluten-free rice bread or sprouted grain bread
- 3 whole eggs
- 1 Weight-Gainer Protein Drink (See page 173)

LUNCH
- Large green salad
- 2 tbs salad dressing of choice, sugar-free and low-carb
- 1 large yam or sweet potato
- 4-6 oz lean beef, chicken, fish, or turkey
- 1 Weight-Gainer Protein Drink (See page 173)

DINNER
- 1 cup steamed vegetables, topped with 1 oz cheese
- 1 baked yam, sweet potato, baking potato, or 2 cups brown rice
- 1 tbs butter or sour cream
- 4-6 oz lean beef, chicken, fish, or turkey
- 1 Weight-Gainer Protein Drink (See page 173)

I recommend consuming at least 1/2 gallon of water each day.

For supplements, I recommend daily:
- 1 multi-vitamin and mineral packet (comprehensive formula)
- 6 desiccated liver tablets (1500 mg each)
- 4-8 tbs golden flax seeds (ground fine)
- 300 mg Vitamin C from acerola berry powder (3 times daily)
- 1500 mg free-form L-Lysine (500 mg at each meal)
- 1-2 tbs sweet dairy whey
- 4-6 tbs whey or egg white protein (avoid soy protein)
- 4-8 tbs dried sweet potato cereal (or powder)

Part Two: The Cutting Phase
How to get your body fat down to 5% or less without sacrificing your hard-earned muscle.

Once you have been training with weights for several years and have gained all the mass you can by utilizing my bulking phase program, you may desire to trim down to get the actual "look" of a bodybuilder. I estimate hundreds of thousands of body-builders each year fail to gain the size they desire because they do not lay the foundation needed by starting with the bulking phase. The latest fashion in bodybuilding is to stay lean year-round and to try to gain muscle while still keeping your abs. Sorry to disappoint you, but only the genetically gifted and those on anabolic steroids can achieve this feat. We, mere mortals, must first bulk up for 12 to 24 months and then follow a cutting phase diet to get lean.

The secret to getting lean is to carb-deplete and carb-load in a unique rotating cycle that I have developed. Also remember, you will be getting smaller on this phase of the program. When I say smaller, I mean smaller in overall size—but not in muscle size. In fact, if you do the cutting phase properly, you should retain almost 100% of the muscle mass that you built prior to the cutting phase.

Some bodybuilders have psychological problems when they

start to trim down because they are fearful of losing size. Some bodybuilders fear being "small," so cutting back is hard for them. These bodybuilders usually prefer to stay bigger, rounder, and smoother. But, in reality, they are really not bodybuilders. They are weightlifters. The true bodybuilder is LEAN and usually maintains 8% body fat or less (except during bulking phases). Weightlifters, power lifters, and strength athletes are SMOOTH and carry 10% or more body fat year-round.

Preparing for a contest is a great goal and vehicle for getting in top condition. Contests give you a specific goal, date, and time to peak and look your absolute best. Preparing for a bodybuilding show also allows you to become more mentally disciplined, which can enhance all other aspects of your life.

It is ideal to begin a cutting phase for a contest 90 days prior to the event if you have 12% body fat or less and 120 days if you have approximately 15% body fat at the onset. If your body fat is higher than 15%, then you have not bulked up properly, and you must adjust your diet by limiting your calories and carbohydrate intake to reduce your body fat level to 15% or less.

Your cutting phase diet will look something like the following (please adjust calories according to your personal needs).

NOTE: If you are lactose intolerant, take a lactase enzyme when consuming milk, sweet dairy whey, or any dairy products that contain lactose.

DAYS 1 and 2 (Low-carb days)

Upon rising: 12 oz water with juice of ½ lemon (or lime) or 1½ tsp acerola berry powder *and* ½ tsp granulated stevia powder.

BREAKFAST

CHOICE #1:
(Protein drink)

- 16 oz water
- 3-4 tbs low-carb whey or egg white protein powder
- 1 tbs sweet dairy whey (to feed lactobacteria)
- 6 strawberries, fresh or frozen OK
- 1 tsp granulated stevia powder
- 2-4 tbs golden flax seed, ground fine

Mix ALL ingredients in blender until creamy smooth.

CHOICE #2:
2 low-carb protein bars (natural ingredients, no refined sugar)

CHOICE #3:
5 egg whites, 1 yolk
1 apple or orange
4 oz lean beef patty or 4 oz skinless chicken breast

Supplements to consume with breakfast: 1 multi-vitamin/mineral packet, 300 mg Vitamin C (from 1½ tsp acerola berry powder mixed in water), and 500 mg free-form L-Lysine.

LUNCH

CHOICE #1:
- 4 cups mixed vegetable salad
- 1 tbs dressing of choice
- 5-8 oz lean meat of choice
- 1-2 cups steamed vegetables

CHOICE #2:
- Protein drink—same as today's protein drink, CHOICE #1

CHOICE #3:
- 2 low-carb protein bars (natural ingredients, no refined sugar)

Supplements to consume with lunch: 6 desiccated liver tablets, 2 EPA-rich fish oil capsules, 300 mg Vitamin C (from 1½ tsp acerola berry powder mixed in water), and 500 mg free-form L-Lysine.

The Fat Burning Diet

DINNER

Repeat today's LUNCH menu (including supplements).

DAY 3 (High-carb day)

Upon rising: 12 oz water with juice of ½ lemon (or lime) or 1½ tsp acerola berry powder *and* ½ tsp granulated stevia powder.

BREAKFAST

CHOICE #1:
(Protein drink)
- 16 oz water or nonfat plain milk
- 1 tbs whey or egg white protein
- 4-6 tbs dried sweet potato cereal (or powder)
- 1 tbs sweet dairy whey
- 2 tbs golden flax seed, ground fine

Mix in blender until creamy smooth.

CHOICE #2:
- 3 egg whites, 1 yolk
- 2 cups hash brown potatoes
- 1 banana

CHOICE #3:
- 2 high-carb energy bars (natural ingredients, no refined sugar) *or* 1 large bowl cream of rice cereal topped with nonfat milk and 1 tbs real maple syrup

CHOICE #4:
- 3 servings in-season fresh fruit (your choice)

Supplement to consume with breakfast: 1 multi-vitamin/mineral packet.

LUNCH

CHOICE #1:
- 1-2 baked potatoes or sweet potatoes
- 2-3 oz lean meat of choice
- 3 cups mixed vegetable salad
- 1 tbs dressing of choice

CHOICE #2:
- 2 cups brown rice
- 1 cup steamed vegetables
- 2-3 oz lean meat of choice

CHOICE #3:
- High-carb protein drink—same as today's breakfast protein drink, CHOICE #1

CHOICE #4:
- 1-2 high-carb energy bars (natural ingredients, no refined sugar)

DINNER

Repeat today's LUNCH menu (including supplements).

Repeat the cycle eating two low-carb days followed by one high-carb day until your body fat is as low as you desire.

CUTTING PHASE GUIDELINES:

1. **Perform 30 minutes** of cardiovascular training every other day. No more, no less.

2. **Be consistent with your diet**—eat two days of low-carb meals followed by one full day of high-carb meals. Repeat the cycle.

3. **If you lose weight too quickly, increase calories slightly**. If you

are not losing fast enough, cut calories slightly.

4. **Stop ALL training** 5 days out from the show.

5. **Limit salt and dairy intake** at 2 days out.

6. **Drink distilled water** at 2 days out. Consume ½ to 1 gallon both days.

7. **If your show is on Saturday**, carb-deplete on Tuesday and Wednesday. Then carb-load for TWO full days on Thursday and Friday.

8. **On the day of the event**, eat light and consume a balance of protein to carbs at **each meal** to maintain your energy levels and glycogen levels.

If you follow the above-referenced program consistently, you will step on stage in the best shape of your life. Your body will be lean, vascular, and strong. The secret is to consistently carb-deplete and carb-load, as outlined.

For more information on bodybuilding, please refer to my book, *Secrets to Successful Bodybuilding Without Steroids* available on-line at www.JayRobb.com.

> "If you really want to be happy,
> nobody can stop you."
> —Sister Mary Tricky

Chapter 19
Delicious Fat Burning Recipes

"Burning fat is as refreshing as a cool
breeze through a camel's knees."
—The Author

Nothing is more delightful than creating delicious meals from scratch—using whole foods that form a combination of nutrients that, once eaten, will allow your body to access fat for fuel. It allows you to have your cake and eat it, too! (Sorry, no cake on *this* diet. Instead, we have Banana Dream Pies!) It is exciting to know that these scrumptious meals are also energizing.

Organization is key when you are cooking. I like to have my pantry and kitchen cabinets stocked full with the essentials so I can avoid unnecessary trips to the store. There is nothing more frustrating than getting halfway through a recipe only to find that you are missing one or two ingredients.

I have prepared a partial list of items you will need in your new FAT BURNING KITCHEN:

- ☐ 8-inch Teflon skillet
- ☐ 12-inch Teflon skillet
- ☐ sauce pan
- ☐ colander (for rinsing)
- ☐ set of measuring spoons
- ☐ measuring cup—one- or two-cup capacity
- ☐ sharp knife
- ☐ cutting board
- ☐ blender

The Fat Burning Diet

- ☐ mixing bowls
- ☐ several large spoons
- ☐ mixer with rotating blades
- ☐ potholders
- ☐ muffin pan
- ☐ aluminum foil
- ☐ toothpicks
- ☐ rubber spatula
- ☐ cheese grater

I have also prepared a FAT BURNING DIET SHOPPING LIST:

Meat *(the leanest hormone-free cuts available)*
___ *chicken breasts*
___ *fresh fish*
___ *7% lean ground sirloin*
___ *salmon fillets*
___ *tuna—no-salt, water-packed*
___ *turkey breast, sliced from deli*

Eggs *(from chickens not given exogenous hormones)*
___ *egg whites*
___ *whole chicken eggs*

Dairy *(from cows not given exogenous hormones)*
___ *cheese, low-fat*
___ *cottage cheese, low-fat*
___ *heavy whipping cream*
___ *mozzarella cheese, low-fat*
___ *plain yogurt, nonfat*
___ *real butter, unsalted*
___ *sour cream, low-fat*
___ *string cheese*

Vegetables (organically grown whenever possible)
___ acorn squash
___ baby carrots, peeled
___ broccoli
___ butternut squash
___ cabbage
___ carrots
___ cauliflower
___ celery
___ cilantro
___ cucumber
___ escarole
___ green onion
___ lettuce
___ mushrooms
___ peppers (all varieties)
___ potatoes (all varieties)
___ radishes
___ spinach
___ sweet potatoes
___ tomatoes
___ yams
___ zucchini

Fresh Fruit (organically grown whenever possible)
___ apples
___ avocados
___ bananas
___ blueberries
___ cantaloupe
___ grapefruit
___ grapes
___ honeydew
___ papaya
___ peaches
___ pineapples
___ plums
___ mangos

The Fat Burning Diet

___ oranges
___ strawberries
___ tangerines
___ watermelons

Raw Nuts & Seeds *(organic and shelled)*
___ almonds
___ golden flax seeds
___ filberts (hazelnuts)
___ macadamia nuts
___ pecans
___ walnuts

Fats & Oils
___ extra virgin olive oil
___ flax seed oil

Grains *(organically grown whenever possible)*
___ brown rice
___ millet
___ popcorn
___ rice cereal
___ sweet potato cereal (nuggets)

Breads & Pasta *(organically grown whenever possible)*
___ 100% flourless sprouted no-salt bread
___ corn pastas
___ corn tortillas
___ rice pastas
___ frozen waffles—FREE of gluten, wheat, dairy, and egg

Specialty Food Items & Supplements
___ agave

___ *egg white protein*
___ *protein bars (low-carb, natural ingredients)*
___ *soy protein (for vegans)*
___ *stevia, granulated powder*
___ *sparkling water*
___ *sweet potato nuggets or powder*
___ *tofu*
___ *tortilla chips, baked*
___ *whey protein*

Condiments, Herbs & Spices
___ *barbecue sauce*
___ *basil flakes*
___ *basil, fresh*
___ *black pepper*
___ *Bragg's Liquid Aminos (natural soy sauce)*
___ *cayenne pepper*
___ *cinnamon*
___ *herb teas*
___ *Knox, unflavored gelatin*
___ *maple syrup*
___ *no-salt mustard*
___ *nutmeg*
___ *oregano flakes*
___ *pasta sauce—no-salt, low-fat*
___ *Red Zinger herb tea*
___ *Rosemary flakes*
___ *salt substitute, potassium-based*

My experience in the kitchen creating recipes for this book was awesome. Every recipe in this book is delicious, healthy, and easy to prepare. It gives me great pleasure to now share them with you. *Giving* really is one of the greatest pleasures in life!

NOTE: Each recipe is presented to you under a heading that suggests the meal it represents. However, feel free to indulge in any of the meals or recipes whenever your taste buds and/or schedule so obliges. Omelets for dinner and a protein drink for lunch is quite typical in my personal menu plan. To achieve maximum fat burning results, each recipe may be combined with other foods to form a complete meal that contains ample protein and friendly fats and is limited in carbohydrate. All protein drink recipes are already balanced and categorized for your convenience.

Main dishes may be served with a salad and a small piece of low-carbohydrate fruit to form the proper fat burning balance. Recipes suggest serving sizes are for an active medium-size person. Adjust the portions to suit your own caloric needs.

These Fat Burning Recipes Are Fun and Easy to Prepare!

Do not presume that these special fat burning recipes can only be prepared by an experienced chef or homemaker. In fact, a bachelor or rookie to a kitchen will have absolutely no problem whipping together these simple recipes.

Feel free to enjoy yourself as you dance through the kitchen—tossing salads, buzzing blenders, and creating triglyceride-torching masterpieces. Have no fear...once you adapt to the basics of The Fat Burning Diet, you will be able to create *your own* special dishes.

And now for the moment you have all been waiting for... Drum roll, please!

LOW-CARB RECIPES

Cheese Omelet
(Serves 1)

PER SERVING:
Protein 29g
Fat 15g

Carbohydrate 3g
Calories 268

INGREDIENTS:
3 egg whites, 1 yolk
2 oz lite mozzarella cheese, grated

Preheat 8-inch Teflon skillet over medium-low heat. Crack both eggs in bowl, and whip with fork until blended smooth. Pour eggs into heated Teflon pan. Then tilt pan until eggs cover pan evenly. When eggs are solid, sprinkle grated cheese on half of eggs, and fold other half of eggs on top of this. Slide half circle omelet onto plate, and serve with fresh salsa or your favorite pasta sauce.

Turkey Breast Omelet
(Serves 1)

PER SERVING:
Protein 46g
Fat 21g
Carbohydrate 2g
Calories 393

INGREDIENTS:
3 egg whites, 1 yolk—cracked in bowl and whipped with fork
3 oz turkey breast, cooked and sliced
1 green onion, chopped
1 tsp olive oil
1 oz lite mozzarella cheese, grated

In 8-inch Teflon pan, sauté olive oil, green onion, and turkey breast on low-medium heat for 2 minutes—until onion is just barely crisp. Pour eggs into Teflon skillet, and tilt until eggs cover entire pan surface. Cook just until eggs become solid. Sprinkle omelet with grated cheese. Then fold in half, and slide onto plate. Top with salsa or thin slices of fresh tomato.

The Fat Burning Diet

Spinach Omelet
(Serves 1)

PER SERVING:
Protein 30g
Fat 15g
Carbohydrate 8g
Calories 287

INGREDIENTS:
3 egg whites, 1 yolk—cracked in bowl and whipped
3 large spinach leaves, washed and chopped
2 oz lite mozzarella cheese, grated
½ small white onion, chopped fine
1 tsp olive oil
1 clove fresh garlic, chopped

Place olive oil, onion, and garlic in 8-inch Teflon skillet. Sauté until onion begins to brown. Pour eggs into pan, and tilt pan to spread eggs evenly. Place spinach on top of eggs, and cover pan. When eggs are solid, sprinkle omelet with grated cheese, and fold in half.

Slide it from the pan onto a plate, and enjoy!

Hot Diggidy Dogger (my son's favorite)
(Serves 1)

PER SERVING:
Protein 23g
Fat 21g
Carbohydrate 2g
Calories 295

INGREDIENTS:
2 egg whites, 1 yolk—cracked in bowl (avoid breaking yolk)
2 Shelton's brand turkey or chicken hot dogs

Place sliced hot dogs in low-medium heated Teflon skillet, and cook until lightly browned and warmed. Gently slide eggs onto hot dogs, and tilt pan until egg whites cover all hot dog slices. Cover and cook until egg whites are solid and yolks are still runny (sunny-side up). Carefully loosen eggs from pan with Teflon spatula, and slide onto plate.

Top with salsa, avocado slices, and chopped green onion, if desired.

Tune-A-Omelet Supreme
(Serves 1)

PER SERVING:
Protein 42g
Fat 15g
Carbohydrate 4g
Calories 328

INGREDIENTS:
4 egg whites, 2 yolks—beaten together in bowl
½ can (3¼-oz) water-packed tuna—drained and chopped
1 tsp lecithin granules
1 green onion, chopped
1 clove garlic, chopped
¼ cup pure water

In 8-inch Teflon skillet, sauté onions and garlic in ¼-cup water on low-to-medium heat. Add beaten eggs, and sprinkle with lecithin granules and chopped tuna. Cover and cook just until eggs become firm.

Fold over, slide omelet onto plate, and serve.

Turkey Time & Sunshine
(Serves 1)

PER SERVING:
Protein 36g
Fat 19g
Carbohydrate 2g
Calories 335

INGREDIENTS:
4 egg whites, 2 yolks
2 oz turkey, cooked and sliced thin
1 tsp olive oil

Place olive oil and turkey in Teflon skillet, and sauté for a few minutes. Crack eggs into pan, discard 2 yolks, and be careful not to break remaining 2 yolks. Cover pan, and cook until whites are solid and yolks are runny (sunny-side up).

Blueberry Power Pancakes
(Serves 2-3)
Recipe makes approximately eight 4-inch pancakes.

PER SERVING (Two pancakes contain):
Protein 25g
Fat 16g
Carbohydrate 14g
Calories 281

INGREDIENTS:
9 egg whites
3 egg yolks
2 tsp lecithin granules
3 tbs olive oil or sunflower oil

¼-½ cup pure water
4 tbs egg white protein (natural vanilla flavor)
1 tsp baking powder
½ cup soy flour
½ cup blueberries, fresh or frozen OK

Using an electric beater, mix all wet ingredients in first bowl. Place all dry ingredients in second bowl, and stir with spoon or fork until well blended. Mix dry ingredients with wet ingredients, and blend with electric beaters until creamy smooth—adding water gradually, as needed, until mixture is very thick but can still be poured. Add grated apple and blueberries, and stir with spoon until evenly mixed. For an occasional treat, add small handful of shelled English walnuts or raw sunflower seeds.

Cook in Teflon pan over medium heat just as you would a regular pancake. These delicious pancakes rise high and taste better than any regular pancake I have ever experienced. (My son Angelo loves them and requests "dear old dad" to make them every week.) These pancakes may be topped with 1 tablespoon nonfat plain yogurt and/or a few sliced strawberries. Flax seed oil, a little "real" butter, or lecithin granules may also be used as a delicious and healthy topping.

To bake **Blueberry Muffins**, simply place 3-4 heaping tablespoons of pancake recipe (for each muffin) in Teflon-coated muffin (cupcake) pan. Spray pan with light oil to ensure no sticking occurs while baking. Bake at 375°F/190°C for approximately 15-18 minutes—until top of muffins are brown and toothpick comes clean after poking the center.

Cabbage Patch Power
(Serves 1)

PER SERVING:
Protein 36g
Fat 2g
Carbohydrate 6g
Calories 187

INGREDIENTS:
½ head green cabbage, sliced very thin
3 red radishes, sliced thin
2 green onions, chopped
5 oz turkey breast, cooked and diced

Place sliced cabbage on plate, and spread evenly. Add radishes and green onions to create a colorful dish. Top with diced turkey, and cover with 1 to 2 tablespoons of your favorite salad dressing.

Taco Salad
(Serves 1)

PER SERVING:
Protein 36g
Fat 19g
Carbohydrate 14g
Calories 428

INGREDIENTS:
¼ head lettuce, chopped or sliced thin
1 cup green cabbage, sliced thin
½ tomato, diced
10 cilantro leaves, pluck leaves from stems
¼ medium-size ripe avocado, peeled and sliced thin
4 oz extra lean (7% fat) ground beef, browned in skillet
½ yellow onion, chopped
1 tsp chili powder

Brown ground beef with onion and chili powder. Spread lettuce and cabbage evenly on large plate. Cover lettuce and cabbage with ground beef mixture. Add chopped tomato and cilantro leaves. Top with fresh salsa and avocado slices. (This is one of my favorite dinners!)

Tuna Salad Supreme
(Serves 1)

PER SERVING:
Protein 44g
Fat 17g
Carbohydrate 4g
Calories 354

INGREDIENTS:
6-oz can water-packed no-salt tuna, drained
1 green onion, chopped
2 red radishes, sliced
1 stalk celery, chopped
1 tbs mustard, no-salt
1 tbs olive oil or flax oil
1/8 tsp cayenne pepper
1 parsley sprig

Place tuna in medium-size bowl, and cover with onion, radishes, celery, oil, and cayenne pepper. Mix together well, and serve with parsley sprig.

Maxi-Burn Meat Loaf
(Serves 6)

PER SERVING:
Protein 47g
Fat 16g
Carbohydrate 5g
Calories 395

The Fat Burning Diet

INGREDIENTS:
2 lb extra lean (7%) ground beef
2 tbs chili powder
4 egg whites, 1 yolk
2 cloves garlic, diced
1 large onion, chopped
1 tbs parsley flakes
4 tbs tomato paste

Preheat oven to 375°F/190C°. Place ingredients, except tomato paste, in bowl and mix. Place meat loaf in oiled baking dish, and cover with tomato paste. Bake 50-60 minutes.

Green Beaner
(Serves 2)

PER SERVING:
Protein 65g
Fat 16g
Carbohydrate 16g
Calories 425

INGREDIENTS:
3 cups fresh green beans—end-clipped and cut in half
¼ cup raw almonds, chopped in blender
12 oz turkey breast, cooked and chopped
2 oz lite mozzarella cheese, grated

Steam green beans for 10-15 minutes—until tender. Place cooked beans, evenly divided, on two plates. Cover with almonds and cheese. Toss lightly and serve.

Chicken Breast Bonanza
(Serves 6)

PER SERVING:
Protein 47g
Fat 8g
Carbohydrate 2g
Calories 277

INGREDIENTS:
2 lb boneless, skinless chicken breasts
1 tbs parsley flakes
1 clove garlic, chopped
1 tbs olive oil
1 medium onion, sliced thin
½ lemon—sliced thin, no seeds

Preheat oven to 375°F/190°C. Place chicken breasts in deep baking dish. Cover chicken with olive oil, parsley flakes, garlic, and onion slices. Top with lemon slices, cover dish with aluminum foil, and bake for 30-40 minutes.

Navel Orange Roughy
(Serves 6)

PER SERVING:
Protein 38g
Fat 13g
Carbohydrate 2g
Calories 260

INGREDIENTS:
2 lbs orange roughy, thawed if you purchase your fish frozen
1 tsp garlic powder
½ navel orange, sliced
1 tbs parsley flakes
1 tbs olive oil

Place orange slices in broiling pan lined with aluminum foil. Place orange roughy on top of orange slices. Cover fish with olive oil, and sprinkle with parsley and garlic. Broil for 12-15 minutes, paying attention not to overcook.

Shrimp-dilly-ishuss!
(Serves 3)

PER SERVING:
Protein 43g
Fat 15g
Carbohydrate 24g
Calories 397

INGREDIENTS:
1 lb small frozen shrimp, cleaned
1 lb green beans, fresh or frozen OK
½ lb green peas, fresh or frozen OK
2 tbs olive oil
2 hard-boiled eggs
1 small onion
4 cloves fresh garlic
1/8 tsp black pepper
1/8 tsp cumin
½ tsp basil

In large pan, steam green beans and peas—until tender. In non-stick skillet, add 1 tablespoon olive oil and garlic, and sauté for one minute over medium heat. Add frozen shrimp and diced onion. Turn up heat slightly. Do not cover pan. Add black pepper, sea salt, cumin, dried oregano, and basil. Add remaining tablespoon of olive oil, and continue turning and cooking shrimp—until lightly browned. Place cooked green beans and peas in large serving bowl, and top with cooked shrimp. Toss lightly and then top with chopped hard-boiled eggs.

HIGH-CARB RECIPES

Fat Burning Yam & Eggs
(Serves 1)

PER SERVING:
Protein 22g
Fat 10g
Carbohydrate 31g
Calories 305

INGREDIENTS:
4 egg whites
1 whole egg
1 medium-size Garnett yam
1 tsp olive oil (to coat yam and skillet)
1 oz mozzarella cheese, grated
2 cherry tomatoes, washed

Wash yam, coat lightly with olive oil, wrap in aluminum foil, and bake 400°F/205°C for an hour or more—until soft to the touch. Remove from oven, and cool. Cut into ½-inch slices, and use as instructed below.

In olive oil-coated non-stick skillet heated to medium-low, place whole egg and egg whites. Cover with lid, and cook slowly—until whites are solid and yolk is lightly cooked but still slightly runny. Slide cooked eggs onto large plate, and decorate by placing yam slices in semi-circle around eggs. Sprinkle cheese on top, and garnish with fresh parsley and cherry tomatoes.

Dig into this fabulous fat burning breakfast that is loaded with all the nutrition you need for a power-charged day!

The Fat Burning Diet

Basic Brown Rice
(Serves 4)

PER SERVING:
Protein 4g
Fat 3g
Carbohydrate 36g
Calories 214

INGREDIENTS:
1 cup brown rice
2 cups pure water
2 tsp olive oil or real butter—not margarine

Place water, oil, and rice in large saucepan, and bring to a rapid boil. Reduce to low heat, cover, and cook for 35-45 minutes—until rice is fluffy and thoroughly cooked.

Yams & Sweet Potatoes
(Serves 2-3)

PER SERVING:
Protein 4g
Fat 12g
Carbohydrate 63g
Calories 369

INGREDIENTS:
4 large yams or sweet potatoes
1 tbs real butter
4 pieces aluminum foil

Preheat oven to 375°F/190°C. Lightly coat each potato with butter, and pierce with fork to break skin (this prevents them from exploding). Wrap each sweet potato with aluminum foil. Bake for 60 minutes or longer—until each sweet potato is soft to the touch and well cooked. Large potatoes may require up to

1½ hours of cooking time.

The butter and aluminum foil seal in the moisture and make the skin (where a great deal of nutrients are housed) soft and tender so you can eat the potato—skin and all!

Butter-Baked Potatoes
(Serves 2-3)

PER SERVING:
Protein 12g
Fat 12g
Carbohydrate 134g
Calories 682

INGREDIENTS:
4 large Russet baking potatoes—washed, not peeled
1 tbs real butter (not margarine)
4 pieces aluminum foil (large enough to wrap each potato)

Preheat oven to 375°F/190°C. Lightly coat each potato with butter, and pierce with fork to break skin (this prevents them from exploding). Wrap each potato with aluminum foil. Bake for 60 minutes or longer—until each potato is soft to the touch and well cooked. Large potatoes may require up to 1½ hours of cooking time.

The butter and aluminum foil seal in the moisture and make the skin (where a great deal of nutrients are housed) soft and tender so you can eat the potato—skin and all!

Baked Squash
(Serves 1)

PER SERVING:
Protein 4g
Fat 2g
Carbohydrate 117g
Calories 502

INGREDIENTS:
1 butternut squash or variety of choice
1 cup pure water

Preheat oven to 375°F/190°C. Cut squash in half, and scoop out seeds. Place each half face down on baking pan that is covered with aluminum foil and misted with olive oil. Fill pan with water, and place in oven. Bake for 50 to 80 minutes, depending on size of squash. The squash is ready when it is very soft to the touch.

Chicken Tacos
(Serves 1)

PER SERVING:
Protein 35g
Fat 23g
Carbohydrate 53g
Calories 544

INGREDIENTS:
1 chicken breast—cooked and sliced thin
4 corn tortillas
½ cup cilantro leaves
½ small onion, chopped
½ ripe Haas avocado—peeled, pitted, and cubed
4 tbs salsa

One at a time, place each tortilla in skillet heated to medium-high, and cook until very warm. Fill warm tortilla with chicken, onion, cilantro, and avocado. Do the same with each tortilla.

Quick Tofu Stir Fry
(Serves 2)

PER SERVING:
Protein 27g
Fat 19g
Carbohydrate 64g
Calories 534

INGREDIENTS:
1-lb package firm tofu, drained and cut into ½-inch cubes
2 tsp olive oil
1 package oriental vegetables, frozen
2 tsp Bragg's Liquid Aminos (natural soy sauce)
1 tsp curry powder
1 small piece fresh ginger, grated
2 cups cooked brown rice (See page 198)
3 oz red cabbage (optional garnish)
1 small carrot (optional garnish)
3 orange slices (optional garnish)

This recipe requires use of two non-stick skillets. In first skillet heated to medium-high and lightly coated with olive oil, place tofu—and cook lightly until browned, stirring occasionally. Remove from heat. In second skillet heated to medium-high and lightly coated with olive oil, place oriental vegetables, curry powder, and ginger—and cook until tender and soft. To this, add cooked tofu and Bragg's Liquid Aminos—and stir lightly until veggies and tofu are well combined. Remove from heat, and serve on plate.

To make this dish look even *more* mouthwatering, garnish plate with thinly sliced red cabbage, grated carrot, and a slice of orange.

Sweet Potato Pancakes
(Serves 3)

PER SERVING:
Protein 17g
Fat 7g
Carbohydrate 64
Calories 389

INGREDIENTS:
¾ cup brown rice flour
¾ cup dried sweet potato cereal (yam nuggets)
1 tsp aluminum-free baking powder
2 tbs egg white protein powder (vanilla flavor)
1 tbs rice bran
1¾ cups water or nonfat milk
1 tbs olive oil

Begin with two bowls. Mix dry ingredients in first bowl, and wet ingredients in second bowl. Pour bowl of dry ingredients into second bowl of wet ingredients—stir until mixed completely. To cook, pour approximately ¼ cup batter into non-stick medium-heated skillet, and cook until brown on bottom. Flip and brown other side.

When cooked on both sides, transfer each pancake to a plate, and top lightly with real maple syrup.

SPECIALTY SIDE DISHES

Turkey Roll
(Serves 1)

PER SERVING:
Protein 11g
Fat 5g

Carbohydrate 2g
Calories 93

INGREDIENTS:
1 slice turkey breast (from deli case)
1 oz piece string cheese

Lay slice of turkey flat on plate. Place string cheese sideways at one end of turkey slice, and roll up. Eat *as is*.

Protein Peanut Butter
(Serves 1)

PER SERVING:
Protein 23g
Fat 12g
Carbohydrate 12g
Calories 357

INGREDIENTS:
3 tbs natural, unsweetened peanut butter
1 tbs whey protein or egg white protein (vanilla flavor)

Place peanut butter and protein powder in small bowl, and add a few drops of water. Mash together with fork until smooth, adding more water, as needed. May be eaten alone or spread onto celery sticks or other vegetables. Almond butter or any other nut butter may be used in place of peanut butter for variety. The protein powder turns the nut butters into a complete, balanced protein.

The Fat Burning Diet

Power Yogurt
(Serves 1)

PER SERVING:
Protein 36g
Fat 13g
Carbohydrate 24g
Calories 373

INGREDIENTS:
8 oz nonfat plain yogurt
1 tbs flax oil or 2 tbs golden flax seeds (ground fine)
2 tbs whey protein or egg white protein (vanilla flavor)
4 ripe strawberries, sliced

Place all ingredients, except strawberries, in bowl, and stir together until smooth and creamy. Top with sliced strawberries, and enjoy! Fifteen blueberries may also be used for variety. If you are a vegan, use soy yogurt and a vegan protein powder.

Carob Balls
(Makes 4 balls)

PER SERVING (One serving is equivalent to one ball):
Protein 20g
Fat 10g
Carbohydrate 12g
Calories 207

INGREDIENTS:
3 tbs carob powder, raw
3 oz whey protein or egg white protein (vanilla flavor)
1½ tbs olive oil or flax oil
14 English walnut halves
4 tbs seedless raisins
2 tsp rice bran or golden flax seeds—ground fine
pure water (as needed)

Place all ingredients, except water, in bowl, and mix thoroughly with fork. Gradually add water, and mix until mixture turns very thick and can be rolled into balls. (For a delicious deep chocolate taste, substitute non-carbohydrate chocolate-flavored egg white protein powder for vanilla-flavored protein powder.)

DELICIOUS PROTEIN DRINKS

All protein drinks must be made with a high-quality egg white or whey protein powder that DOES NOT contain "added" carbohydrate (look for a high-end protein powder that is sugar-free, fat-free, chemical-free and contains "naturally occurring" carbohydrate). When you purchase this basic formula protein powder, read the ingredients disclosure very carefully. If you are a vegan, purchase a vegetable-, rice-, or soy-based protein powder. Be aware of the fact that protein powders containing soy or isolated soy protein can sometimes cause gas and/or indigestion.

Delicious high-carb protein drinks often use bananas and/or a dried sweet potato cereal (yam nuggets).

To mix protein drinks, place ALL ingredients in a blender, and blend until creamy smooth (approximately 45 seconds). It is best to add protein powder *while blending*—to keep it from clumping together. All recipes will produce one serving, unless otherwise stated. Add ice or freeze the fruit if a frosty cold drink is desired. To prevent arthritis and enhance the strength of your joints, tendons, ligaments, and cartilage—try adding (while blending) one tablespoon of an ionic liquid mineral formula and one tablespoon of unsweetened, unflavored gelatin to any of the protein drinks listed. For added FIBER, and to enhance colon activity, add one or two tablespoons of finely ground golden flax seeds.

LOW-CARB PROTEIN DRINKS

Protein Power!

PER SERVING:
Calories 330

INGREDIENTS:
12 oz pure water
1 cup ripe strawberries, fresh or frozen OK
1 tbs flax seed oil or nut butter
2 tbs whey protein or egg white protein (vanilla flavor)

Tropical Treasure

PER SERVING:
Calories 291

INGREDIENTS:
6 oz pure water
½ small papaya
1 tsp lecithin granules or liquid
2 tbs whey protein or egg white protein (vanilla flavor)
½ tsp coconut extract

Inner-G Supreme

PER SERVING:
Calories 386

INGREDIENTS:
3 oz pure water
1 orange, juiced
1 tbs flax seed oil or nut butter
2 tbs whey protein or egg white protein (vanilla flavor)
½ tsp pineapple extract

Instant Breakfast

PER SERVING:
Calories 301

INGREDIENTS:
12 oz pure water
1 cup strawberries
2 tbs whey protein or egg white protein (vanilla flavor)

Fat Burner Supreme

PER SERVING:
Calories 342

INGREDIENTS:
8 oz pure water
1 peach, pitted
1 tbs flax oil or nut butter
3 tbs whey protein or egg white protein (vanilla flavor)
½ cup strawberries

Vanilla I-Scream Delight!
(An occasional treat)

PER SERVING:
Calories 524

INGREDIENTS:
2 oz fresh cream
4 oz pure water
1 ripe banana, frozen
2 tbs whey protein or egg white protein (vanilla flavor)
1 tsp pure vanilla

The Fat Burning Diet

Build-a-Body

PER SERVING:
Calories 537

INGREDIENTS:
8 oz pure water
4 tbs whey protein or egg white protein (vanilla flavor)
1 banana, frozen
1 tsp lecithin, granules or liquid

Famous Banana Delight
(A *Jay's Gym* Classic)

PER SERVING:
Calories 330

INGREDIENTS:
8 oz pure water or nonfat milk
½ banana, frozen OK
1 tbs flax seed oil
2 tbs whey protein or egg white protein (vanilla flavor)

Maxi-Burner

PER SERVING:
Calories 323

INGREDIENTS:
8 oz pure water
1 tsp lecithin, granules or liquid
¼ cup blueberries, frozen
2 tbs whey protein or egg white protein (vanilla flavor)
½ tbs flax oil
½ banana

Bodybuilding "Super Cuts"

PER SERVING:
Calories 356

INGREDIENTS:
12 oz pure water
½ cup frozen strawberries
½ banana
4 tbs whey protein or egg white protein (vanilla flavor)
1 tbs flax oil

Peaches & Cream

PER SERVING:
Calories 343

INGREDIENTS:
6 oz pure water
1 oz heavy cream
1 ripe peach, pitted
2 tbs whey protein or egg white protein (vanilla flavor)

HIGH-CARB PROTEIN DRINKS

Yammer-Jammer

PER SERVING:
Calories 475

INGREDIENTS:
8 oz nonfat milk
2 tbs dried sweet potato cereal (or powder)
1 tbs whey protein or egg white protein (vanilla flavor)
1 tbs golden flax seeds—ground fine

Banana-Slammer

PER SERVING:
Calories 441

INGREDIENTS:
12 oz nonfat milk or pure water
1 ripe banana
2 tbs whey protein or egg white protein (vanilla flavor)
1 tbs peanut butter

PROTEIN DRINKS FOR VEGANS
—Use a low-carb soy protein powder.

Vegan Power!

PER SERVING:
Calories 358

INGREDIENTS:
10 oz pure water
½ banana
¼ cup blueberries
1 tbs flax seed oil
3 tbs soy protein powder (vanilla flavor)

Peachy Lean

PER SERVING:
Calories 361

INGREDIENTS:
10 oz pure water
1 peach, peeled and pitted
1 tbs flax seed oil
3 tbs soy protein powder (vanilla flavor)

Berry Fine!

PER SERVING:
Calories 353

INGREDIENTS:
10 oz pure water
½ cup blueberries
6 strawberries
1 tbs sunflower or flax seed oil
3 tbs soy protein powder (vanilla flavor)

Break Fast

PER SERVING:
Calories 361

INGREDIENTS:
10 oz pure water
1 orange, peeled and seedless
1 tbs flax seed oil
4 strawberries
3 tbs soy protein powder (vanilla flavor)

SPECIALTY RECIPES

Homemade Sauerkraut
(Serves 8)

PER SERVING:
Calories 10

INGREDIENTS:
2 heads green cabbage
1 earthenware crock

Cut cabbage into very thin strips, and place in crock until you

The Fat Burning Diet

have a layer about 3 inches deep. Tamp this down very well with a *clean* 2 x 4 piece of wood (cut the length of a rolling pin). Then add the rest of the cabbage—doing the same—until cabbage is pressed in tight. There must be no air present between the cabbage pieces!

Cover this with clean piece of cheesecloth and thick paper plate. Place 10-pound weight or one-gallon jug of water on top of crock pot to give mixture constant pressure. Place crock somewhere warm (at least 70°F/21°C), and leave undisturbed for 7 to 10 days. When sauerkraut is ready, divide evenly (including the juice), and refrigerate in glass jars for storage.

This recipe is even easier if made in a Japanese pickle press that may be purchased from your local health food store.

FRESH SALSA
(Serves 6)

PER SERVING:
Protein 2g
Fat 5g
Carbohydrate 6g
Calories 71

INGREDIENTS:
3 tbs flax seed oil
3 tomatoes, chopped fine
4 sprigs fresh cilantro
½ medium onion, chopped
1 green onion, chopped
1 small jalapeno pepper, chopped
½ cup tomato sauce, sugar- and salt-free

Place ALL ingredients in large bowl, and mix together with large spoon. If you like your salsa hot, then use 2 jalapeno peppers.

DELICIOUS DESSERTS

—These fun foods are ideal for special occasions, the holidays, or your once-a-week FREE MEAL.

Banana Dream Pie
(Serves 8)

PER SERVING:
Protein 16g
Fat 15g
Carbohydrate 16g
Calories 262

Approximate Preparing Time:
15 minutes

Utensils Needed:
1 blender
1 small saucepan
1 measuring cup
1 set measuring spoons

Filling:
1½ cups water
3 packages unflavored gelatin
3 ripe bananas
6 tbs whey protein or egg white protein (vanilla flavor)
1 pint half and half
1 tsp vanilla extract

Crust:
1 cup raw almonds (or English walnuts)

Place ½ cup of room temperature water in saucepan, and sprinkle with gelatin. Let stand one minute at room temperature—then stir, until dissolved, using low heat. Set this aside. In blender, add 1 cup raw almonds, and blend on low until chopped fine. Pour into bowl and set aside.

Using same blender, add remaining cup of water, bananas, protein powder, half and half, vanilla, and ½ cup of dissolved gelatin (that you set aside). Blend for 45-60 seconds—until smooth. Lightly coat a 9-inch pie pan with flax seed oil, and pour above-blended mixture into pan.

Cover with clear plastic wrap, and place in freezer for 1 hour—or in refrigerator for 3 hours—until gelatin is firm and set. Once set, top with chopped almonds, spreading them evenly across top of the pie. Cut and serve.

This truly is a dream pie that will not give you a sugar rush. For a holiday treat, substitute 8 ounces of cream cheese for the half and half to make a rich **Banana Cheese Cake**. Cover this special holiday pie, after it has set, with fresh whipped cream (no sugar), and sprinkle with a few tablespoons of chopped almonds.

Cottage Cheese Supreme
(Serves 1)

PER SERVING:
Protein 26 g
Fat 18 g
Carbohydrate 19 g
Calories 210

INGREDIENTS:
6 oz low-fat cottage cheese
½ cup strawberries, sliced
4 shelled walnut halves

Place cottage cheese in bowl. Cover with strawberries and nuts.

Cinnamon Apple Delight
(Serves 1)

PER SERVING:
Protein 26g
Fat 14g
Carbohydrate 19g
Calories 229

INGREDIENTS:
6 oz low-fat cottage cheese
½ apple—peeled, cored, and diced
4 shelled walnut halves
Ground cinnamon

Place cottage cheese in bowl. Cover with apple and walnuts. Sprinkle with cinnamon to taste.

SUPER SALAD DRESSINGS

Mixing Instructions: Place ALL listed ingredients for each recipe into blender, and mix for 30-45 seconds on medium. Store dressings in refrigerator.

One-fourth teaspoon pure sun-dried sea salt may be added to any of the following recipes, if desired.

Italiano Supreme

INGREDIENTS:
½ cup olive oil
½ cup pure water
1 clove garlic, diced
½ lemon, juiced
½ tsp oregano

The Fat Burning Diet

Flax Attack!

INGREDIENTS:
½ cup flax seed oil
½ cup pure water
1 clove garlic, diced
2 tbs raw apple cider vinegar

Creamy Smooth

INGREDIENTS:
¼ cup sunflower oil
¼ cup flax oil
¼ cup water
½ orange, juiced
2 oz cream cheese

Italian Power!

INGREDIENTS:
½ cup olive oil
½ cup pure water
2 cloves garlic
3 tbs apple cider vinegar
¼ tsp black pepper
½ tsp basil

Hot-Cha-Cha!

INGREDIENTS:
½ cup cottage cheese
½ cup flax oil
½ cup pure water
1/8 tsp cayenne pepper
1 clove garlic, diced
¼ tsp ginger powder

Tomato Thyme

INGREDIENTS:
½ cup olive oil
¼ cup pure water
1 ripe tomato, peeled
1 green onion, diced
1 clove garlic, diced
½ tsp thyme

Lemon Basil Pepper

INGREDIENTS:
½ cup flax seed oil
½ cup pure water
Juice from ½ small lemon
½ tsp oregano
½ tsp basil
¼ tsp black pepper

Want More Recipes to Help You Burn Fat Fast?

You will discover 100 more outrageously delicious fat burning recipes in Jay Robb's *Fat Burning Diet Cook Book*, available on-line (www.JayRobb.com), or call 1.877.JAY.ROBB.

"If you become angry with me and I do not get insulted, then the anger falls back on you. You are then the only one who is unhappy, not me. All you have done is hurt yourself. If you want to stop hurting yourself, you must get rid of your anger and become loving instead. When you hate others, you, yourself, become unhappy. But when you love others, everyone is happy."
—Buddha

Chapter 20

Jay's Nutritional
Supplement Suggestions

"When your cup is empty, God will
joyfully fill it to the brim."
—The Author

Nutritional supplements are just that—nutrients that supplement a person's diet. Supplements do not replace foods; they enhance foods and can help correct nutritional deficiencies.

There are literally thousands of nutritional supplements on the market. Vitamins, minerals, herbs, protein powders, carbohydrate drinks, and homeopathic remedies are just a few examples of common nutritional supplements.

There Are No "Magic Pills" that Burn Fat

There are no known supplements that actually burn fat, so don't expect to purchase a bottle of pills that will magically dissolve your fat.

Burning fat is a metabolic process that is triggered by the amount and type of foods you eat, the amount and type of physical activities you are engaged in daily, your body temperature (metabolism), and the balance of essential vitamins and minerals that are present in your body. High-quality protein powders are extremely useful to anyone burning fat because they ensure that fat, not muscle, is being burned. Protein powders should be low in carbohydrate and must be blended according to the recipes listed in Chapter 19.

15 Key Nutritional Supplements

1. **Vitamin C** (from acerola berry powder) and **L-Lysine**
2. **Protein powder** (whey, egg white, or soy)
3. **Golden flax seed** (for fiber and Omega-3 oils)
4. **Sweet dairy whey** (for lactobacteria enhancement)
5. **Protein bars** (nutritious time-saver for meals or snacks)
6. **Dried sweet potato cereal** (tasty complex carb source)
7. **Stevia** (a sweet-tasting herb used in foods)
8. **Desiccated liver** (high in B-vitamins for increased energy)
9. **Chromium** (to help restore insulin's efficiency)
10. **Flax seed oil** (rich source of Omega-3 EFAs)
11. **Liquid ionic minerals** (for overall health and thyroid support)
12. **Multi-vitamin and mineral** (one-a-day packet)
13. **Coral minerals** (a great source of alkaline minerals)
14. **Fish oil capsules** (direct Omega-3 and EPA source)
15. **Digestive enzymes** (to enhance digestive power)

Supplement #1
VITAMIN C AND LYSINE COMBINATION

According to extensive clinical research by Dr. Matthias Rath (who formerly worked with Nobel Prize Winner Dr. Linus Pauling), the intake of Vitamin C and the amino acid L-Lysine form a powerful combination of nutrients that may be our answer to eliminating cancer and heart disease in the world. This is not just speculation. Dr. Rath has clinically proven that— by utilizing key nutrients, especially Vitamin C and L-Lysine— heart disease can be prevented and reversed, and the cell growth of certain types of cancer can be controlled.

Vitamin C

Vitamin C has also been shown to boost the immune system, help build strong bones and teeth, support the adrenal glands, combat stress, slow aging as an antioxidant, help cure drug addiction, protect us from carcinogenic substances, help rebuild collagen, beautify the skin, prevent the common cold, fight viral infections, prevent back injury by supporting the integrity of the disks, and protect us from heavy metal poisoning. And that is just a short list! There are actually well over 150 ailments and conditions that Vitamin C may be beneficial in relieving or curing.

L-Lysine

L-Lysine is an essential amino acid found in complete protein foods. L-Lysine helps build resistance to bacterial invasion, promotes a feeling of well being, and is involved in the body's growth and strength of the immune system.

Suggested Use:

Take 300 mg Vitamin C (from 1½ teaspoon acerola berry powder *and* 500 mg L-Lysine (free-form) **THREE times a day**, preferably with meals. (A therapeutic dose may be double the prevention dose or higher.)

To learn more about Dr. Rath's research and nutritional suggestions, please visit his website at www.dr-rath-research.org.

Supplement #2
PROTEIN POWDERS

The regular use of a high-quality protein powder can save you thousands of hours in the kitchen over the course of your life. You can simply toss into a blender two to four tablespoons of a high-quality low-carb protein powder, 12 ounces of milk or water, some fresh fruit, a tablespoon of flax oil, or 1/2 of an avocado (or a tablespoon or two of almond butter), and you have a meal or snack within seconds. Protein powders offer the convenience of taking in the essential amino acids your body needs at meal times. Having a regular supply of protein can help curb your cravings for sweets and carbs, improve your recovery from exercise, help combat stress, and stabilize your energy and blood sugar levels.

Suggested Use:

Take two or more tablespoons daily of a high-quality protein powder to help meet protein needs.

FIRST CHOICE:
Whey protein
A high-quality protein derived from filtering out most of the lactose in dairy whey. Whey is the liquid that floats to the top during the processing of cheese and cottage cheese. Whey is high in *lactose* (milk sugar). Liquid whey is pressed through a special membrane that removes most of the lactose, leaving a high concentration of whey protein. Crude dairy whey is only about 3% protein before it is filtered. What is left behind, after filtering crude whey, is a very high-quality easy-to-assimilate protein. Whey protein is a dairy product; so if you are allergic to dairy, avoid it.

SECOND CHOICE:
(For those who are sensitive to dairy products.)
Egg white protein
A premium source of protein derived from egg whites that are dried at low heat and made into a powder. Egg white protein is fat-free, dairy-free, and lactose-free, making it ideal for those who have dairy allergies and/or are lactose intolerant. Choose a high-quality egg white protein that does NOT contain any added carbohydrate, sweeteners, or any artificial sweeteners—including acesulfame-K (acesulfame potassium), aspartame, or sucralose.

THIRD CHOICE:
Soy protein
Soy protein can be a fantastic source of protein for individuals who avoid the consumption of ALL animal products (vegans). Be aware that soy protein is not digested well by certain individuals who are sensitive to soy products. While Asians usually tolerate soy very well, very few other ethnic groups do well on soy. Currently, soy products are often valued for their estrogen-enhancing properties (soy is not recommended for men because of this property). In my opinion, for optimum amino acid balance and digestibility, egg white protein and whey protein are still the absolute best protein sources.

Supplement #3
GOLDEN FLAX SEEDS

Flax seeds are nature's perfect source of highly nutritious lignan-rich FIBER. The consumption of high-lignan fiber can help relieve constipation and menopausal hot flashes as well as exhibit anti-cancer, anti-fungal, and anti-viral activity. Research has also shown that flaxseed lignans are changed by the bacteria in the human intestines and can be extremely effective at preventing cancer—especially breast cancer.

The fiber in flax seeds can help stimulate the production of the friendly bacteria in the colon, especially when consumed with nonfat plain yogurt and sweet dairy whey. Because of their rich, creamy taste, golden flax seeds are preferred over traditional brown flax seeds.

Suggested Use:

For additional fiber and essential fatty acids, consume 2-6 tablespoons golden flax seeds (finely ground) daily in protein drinks or with yogurt.

Supplement #4
SWEET DAIRY WHEY

(This is not the same as whey protein.)
Your colon should be in a slightly acidic condition and naturally replete with millions of colonies of *lactobacteria* (your friendly bacteria). Junk-food consumption, the use of antibiotics, the use of laxatives, the use of drugs, and the lack of whole foods and lactose-rich dairy products in one's diet can starve the lactobacteria, causing lactobacteria to die off—thus leading to constipation, diarrhea, gas, bloating, and various colon disorders.

Sweet dairy whey is the liquid that rises to the top during the process of making cheese and cottage cheese. Sweet dairy whey is then spray dried at cold temperatures to form a dry powder. Sweet dairy whey is low in protein and high in *lactose* (milk sugar). Lactose is the primary food for the lactobacteria in your colon, making sweet dairy whey an ideal supplement for feeding the friendly bacteria in your colon.

Suggested Use:
Two tablespoons of sweet dairy whey can be mixed with 8 ounces water or consumed on an empty stomach in the morning. Or it can be mixed with 16 ounces nonfat plain yogurt, taken at breakfast. Fresh fruit, dried sweet potato cereal, and/or finely ground flax seeds may also be mixed with yogurt and whey for a tasty breakfast treat. Two tablespoons of whey should be consumed daily for 30 to 60 days until bowel movements are well formed, nearly odorless, and easy to pass. For maintenance thereafter, two tablespoons of whey taken 3 to 4 times a week may then be necessary to maintain a high population of lactobacteria. Sweet dairy whey can also be taken in water or in a protein drink.

Supplement #5
PROTEIN BARS
Protein bars are a convenient way to access good nutrition and are ideal if your lifestyle is fast-paced. Unfortunately, NOT ALL PROTEIN BARS ARE CREATED EQUAL. In fact, I have taken it upon myself to survey and critique nearly every bar on the market, and I am sad to announce that the majority of bars I found on the market were nothing more than glorified candy bars. Most contained ingredients I would not put in my body, nor would I recommend to clients, family, or friends.

When purchasing a protein bar, make sure that the bar is actually low in carbohydrate. The bar should have the net carbs listed, meaning the carbs it contains that actually impact or raise blood sugar levels. Look for a protein bar with 8 or less grams of net carbs.

AVOID BARS (AND PROTEIN POWDERS)
THAT CONTAIN THE FOLLOWING INGREDIENTS:

- Acesulfame-K
- Acesulfame-potassium
- Artificial colors
- Artificial flavors
- Artificial sweeteners
- Aspartame
- Brown sugar
- Calcium caseinate
- Casein
- Corn syrup
- Corn syrup solids
- Dried cane juice
- Evaporated cane juice
- Fructose
- Glucose polymers
- Gluten
- High-fructose corn sweeteners
- High-fructose corn syrup
- Hydrogenated oils
- Maltitol
- Maltodextrin
- MSG
- Sodium caseinate
- Sorbitol
- Sucralose
- Sugar
- Wheat

If any of the above ingredients are found in a protein bar you are considering buying, I would have to advise you to put the bar down and move away from it quickly. The last thing you need is to put junk in your precious body. As it clearly states in 1 Corinthians 6:19-20, "...the body is a temple of the Spirit," and the last thing you want to do is tear down your temple with a junk-food protein bar. Please beware! There are dozens and dozens of junk-food-laced protein bars on the market, so READ those labels very carefully!

What General Ingredients are Best?

When purchasing a protein bar, look for wholesome ingredients such as "organic" peanut butter, "organic" almond butter, egg white protein, whey protein, and natural fiber from Arabic and guar gums.

What Protein Source is Best?

Egg white protein and whey protein are the two best sources of protein. Many protein bars are made with soy protein (because it is an inexpensive protein). I don't recommend the regular use of soy products or protein except for those of Asian decent and vegan women.

What Sweetener is Best?

Xylitol is one of the best sweeteners on the market and is ideal in a low-carbohydrate protein bar. Xylitol is a sugar alcohol naturally derived from the Birch tree. Hundreds of clinical studies have proven xylitol to be an effective natural sweetener that DOES NOT cause dental caries. In fact, xylitol has been clinically proven to PREVENT tooth decay if consumed daily. Now that is a switch from ordinary white sugar that can rot your teeth faster than just about any other substance known to man. **Xylitol does not significantly raise blood sugar levels—making it safe as a sweetener for diabetics or anyone wishing to control insulin through carbohydrate management.**

A Sample Ingredient List:

(What to look for on the label.) Egg white protein—and/or whey protein—xylitol, organic nut butter, Arabic gum, organic agave, nut pieces, natural flavoring, and guar gum.

Supplement #6
DRIED SWEET POTATO CEREAL (or powder)

On high-carb days, you can meet many of your carbohydrate needs with a fitness cereal made from dried sweet potato pieces. Besides being eaten as a cold cereal with milk, these tasty nuggets can be eaten *as is* for a delicious snack or **mixed into a protein or energy drink**. These nuggets can also be sprinkled over yogurt, soups, salads, hash browns, or other foods to add a unique sweet, crunchy taste. Dried sweet potato bits taste similar to sweet corn flakes. The sweet potato is a slow-releasing complex carbohydrate source that is ideal for carb-loading and glycogen loading.

An Athlete's Dream-Come-True

Dried sweet potato nuggets are also an ideal carb source for endurance athletes, runners, cyclists, triathletes, football players, weightlifters, and strength athletes because the complex carbohydrates can supply a natural source for energy. Currently, most athletes must purchase and use carbohydrate powder made from highly refined cornstarch (called *maltodextrin*) or a s-t-r-e-t-c-h-e-d version of cornstarch (called *glucose polymers*). Using a dried sweet potato product eliminates the need for athletes to consume cheap refined carbohydrates to meet their highly demanding energy needs.

Supplement #7
STEVIA

(Granulated powder is best.)
Stevia is an herb that is native to Paraguay. While stevia is not classed as a sweetener, this unique herb has a pleasant, sweet taste when mixed with foods. Stevia is best consumed as a granulated powder that is blended with *erythritol* (a gluten-free natural fiber from fruits, vegetables, and grains) to make it free-flowing and smooth-tasting.

Suggested Use:

Add small amounts to protein drinks, limeades, lemonade, grapefruit, tea, decaffeinated coffee, baked goods, or foods you wish to make taste sweeter without adding calories or carbohydrate.

Supplement #8
DESICCATED LIVER

Desiccated means "dried"—as in dried beef liver. Why liver? It is a whole food that is high in all the B-vitamins, protein, Vitamin A, and copper. Under stress, I have been known to take up to 15 tablets a day, but my usual dose is four to six daily at low-carb meals. I have used desiccated liver since the mid '70s and truly feel it helped me quickly recover from reactive hypoglycemia and the mental and physical exhaustion that accompanies this disorder.

It is my belief, through research and personal experience, that much of the magical properties of liver are due to the high content of B-vitamins it contains. The Vitamin B Complex consists of eight B-vitamins that are essential and water soluble, meaning they are not stored and must be continuously supplied by one's diet.

The B-vitamins are heavily involved in almost every energy transfer in the human body. Supplementing one's diet with desiccated liver is an excellent means of supplying the body with a natural source of the B-vitamins it needs to stay energized and powerful.

A Vitamin B deficiency may be indicated if a person is tired, irritable, nervous, depressed, or suicidal. A poor appetite, insomnia, constipation, or high cholesterol levels may also indicate a Vitamin B deficiency. Smoking, the consumption of alcohol, stress, sugar consumption, vegetarian diets, and a junk-food diet can all lead to a deficiency of B-vitamins.

Suggested Use:
To combat stress, curb sugar and carbohydrate cravings, and dramatically boost energy levels, take four to six 1500-mg tablets daily—on LOW-CARB DAYS ONLY. Taking desiccated liver on high-carb days may cause gas because it does not digest well with high-carbohydrate foods for some individuals.

Supplement #9
CHROMIUM
(In the form of chromium picolinate, chromium citrate, or chromium polynicotinate.)

Chromium is a trace mineral that affects your energy level in a positive way, aids in blood sugar metabolism, helps you combat stress, helps you control your weight, enhances your fitness potential, can improve your cholesterol level and balance, and can ensure your heart remains healthy.

Suggested Use:
To help restore insulin's efficiency and to stabilize blood sugar levels, an adult should take 600 mcg (three 200-mcg capsules) daily for three months. Take one or two 200-mcg capsules daily for maintenance from then on.

Supplement #10
FLAX SEED OIL
Omega-3 Essential Fatty Acids
To the best of my knowledge, I was the first nutritionist in America to recommend adding flax seed oil to a protein drink so the user could easily obtain Omega-3 essential fats. Omega-3 oils are rich in flax seed oil and in cold-water fish. Omega-3 essential fats can do the following: decrease elevated cholesterol, decrease elevated triglyceride levels, help balance HDL and LDL cholesterol levels, improve oxygen utilization, shorten recovery time from exercise, decrease cravings for fatty foods and sweets, stoke the metabolism, help regulate blood sugar levels, regulate insulin levels, and slow the buildup of lactic acid following exercise.

Flax seeds contain approximately 57% *Omega-3* (linolenic acid) as well as a small amount of *Omega-6* (linoleic acid). Ground flax seeds and flax oil have a delicious nutty taste that greatly enhances the flavor of other foods, especially protein drinks. Because Omega-3 oils are polyunsaturated fats that can oxidize rapidly when exposed to heat, air, and sunlight, do not use flax seed oil for cooking. If you choose to take flax seed oil in capsules, you will need to take approximately nine 1000-mg capsules to equal a tablespoon of fresh oil. Flax seeds and flax seed oil (liquid or capsules) should be refrigerated for a longer shelf life.

Suggested Use:
Consume one tablespoon daily, per 100 pounds of body weight. The oil tastes great in protein drinks or as a salad oil.

Supplement #11
LIQUID IONIC MINERALS
Minerals are critical to good health, and a liquid ionic mineral supplement is an ideal way to ensure you get a hearty supply of major and trace minerals into your body in a form that is easy to assimilate.

Because much of the soil our food is grown on is mineral deficient, the crops may also be low in essential minerals. If the minerals are absent in the food, you can't get them in your body unless you supplement your diet with a high-quality liquid ionic mineral—the ideal way to ensure you are getting a readily available supply of minerals in your body.

Suggested Use:
Consume 1 ounce daily per 100 pounds of body weight. Children may take one teaspoon per 20 pounds of body weight.

Supplement #12
MULIT-VITAMIN AND MINERAL FORMULA
For personal health insurance, it is advisable to make a comprehensive multiple vitamin and mineral part of your daily life. This vitamin and mineral formula should contain the following vitamins: A, D, E, C-Complex (including bioflavanoids), and the entire B-Complex, 360 mg EPA (from fish oil), 240 mg DHA (from fish oil), 500 mg coral calcium, 250 mg coral magnesium as well as a hefty dose of the phytonutrients from fresh fruits and vegetables.

Suggested Use:
Take one packet daily.

Supplement #13
CORAL MINERALS (Also known as "coral calcium.")
Coral minerals are ideal for helping the body maintain its natural pH balance (pH stands for "potential hydrogen"). To test for adequate alkaline mineral reserves in your body, run a strip of pH paper through your urine at midstream, and compare the color of the strip to the chart on the pH paper chart. Daily urine pH should be near 7.0 or slightly higher. A lower reading could indicate a deficiency of alkaline minerals and a lack of vegetables and fruits in the diet. Coral minerals are ideal for helping maintain the proper pH balance of the body. Coral minerals also provide a substantial source for easy-to-absorb calcium and magnesium (at a perfect 2:1 ratio) as well as provide important minerals—including potassium, iron, zinc, iodine, and selenium (plus a whole host of other trace minerals naturally derived from the sea).

Coral minerals are usually harvested from the crystal clear waters near tropical and subtropical islands. Coral minerals are produced in the ocean by the shells and skeletons of reef building (but now defunct) coral.

Maintaining alkaline reserves in the body can also be very important for blood sugar stability by keeping receptor sites sensitized to insulin. This means a diet rich in alkaline minerals could be critical for a diabetic or anyone suffering from hypoglycemia or a blood sugar disorder. The rich and balanced mineral content of coral minerals may improve thyroid function, enhance sleeping, lower high blood pressure, improve ability to relax, combat stress and tension, and help prevent osteoporosis.

Suggested Use:
Take 2000-4000 mg daily.

Supplement #14
FISH OIL CAPSULES

Fish oil capsules are derived from the fat of cold-water fish and are rich in Eicosapentaenoic Acid (EPA), Docosahexaenoic Acid (DHA), and Omega-3 (Linolenic Acid). All of these fatty acids have long carbon chains with multiple double bonds.

Suggested Use:
Take 2 fish oil capsules daily that supply a total of 360 mg EPA and 240 mg DHA.

Supplement #15
DIGESTIVE ENZYMES

Stress, poor food combinations, low body temperatures, high-fat diets, and cooked food can impair your body's ability to digest food properly. Taking a comprehensive digestive enzyme can aid your body in breaking down food so that it can be absorbed by your body and used as nourishment.

Suggested Use:
FULL SPECTRUM ENZYME: Take one or two capsules, as needed, with large meals, free meals, poorly combined meals, or any time a digestive boost is needed.

LACTASE ENZYME (an enzyme used by those who are lactose intolerant): Take one or two capsules when consuming sweet dairy whey or foods containing milk, lactose, or lactose-rich dairy products. I personally take two capsules with my morning dose of sweet dairy whey to ensure I am digesting the lactose properly. A common symptom of lactase deficiency is gas and bloating when dairy products are consumed.

> "All know that the drop merges into the ocean, but few know that the ocean merges into the drop."
> —Kabir

Questions and Answers

"God is the *final answer*."
—The Author

Q. How much weight will I lose on your diet, and at what rate will I lose it?

A. I do not refer to the results attained on this diet as "weight loss" simply because the main purpose of the diet is to burn fat as fuel, thus creating "fat loss," not weight loss. Weight loss could be attributed to water loss, lean muscle loss, and/or fat loss. By restricting carbohydrates and targeting your fat cells as a source of sustainable energy, The Fat Burning Diet stimulates fat loss and absolutely minimizes lean muscle loss, which is just the effect you need for maintaining your precious strength and energy levels. How much fat you can expect to lose and how fast you will lose it really depends upon several factors: a) the amount and type of carbohydrate you intake, b) your present level of fitness, c) the amount of calories you expend each day, and d) the amount of calories you intake each day. My clients usually average 2 pounds of fat loss per week, if they are not physically fit when they begin the diet. For my clients that are already in very good condition, fat loss may be as high as 3 pounds a week, initially.

Q. Is The Fat Burning Diet nutritionally balanced?

A. The Fat Burning Diet is very nutritionally balanced. By includ-

ing whole foods, ample protein, wholesome fats, raw vegetables, raw fruits, raw nuts, and raw seeds, this diet excels in nutritional content. Also, by avoiding poor food combinations (the diet limits protein intake when consumed with starchy foods), you will not only be eating a highly nutritious diet, but your digestion will be greatly improved—thus ensuring that the nutrients are readily available for absorption and utilization within the body.

Q. Why do you keep stressing the importance of avoiding starchy carbohydrates every other day? Will a cup of rice or two pieces of toast really be a problem on low-carb days?

A. Starches and sweets are the two most concentrated forms of carbohydrate that stimulate the maximum need for insulin. To keep glycogen levels from overfilling, starches and sweets are curtailed every other day. This rule must be adhered to, or the diet becomes ineffective.

Q. How can I be sure I'm burning fat while following your diet?

A. It's very simple. Accurately measure your body fat before you begin the diet, and then test it again every 30 days, noting the decrease in body fat percentages. Test your body fat at home with a simple pair of calipers, or have it tested at your local fitness club or doctor's office.

Q. I have been diagnosed with hypoglycemia and am presently eating six small meals a day, consisting mostly of complex carbohydrates and low-fat proteins. The only problem is that I never feel mentally stable and always crave sweets and sugary baked goods. Once I indulge in the forbidden fruit, I become a basket case, feeling weak, shaky, and downright mentally confused. Will The Fat Burning Diet change all this for me? I'm desperate!

A. I have personally experienced the diet you described above, which supposedly controls hypoglycemia, and all it did was keep me in a state of total mental and physical instability. Eating six low-fat meals a day that are rich in complex carbohydrate to control a blood sugar disorder is the exact opposite approach needed for ending this problem. Switch to The Fat Burning Diet principles; eat only three meals a day, as described; and avoid wheat- and gluten-containing grains on the high-carb days. This will take you off the carbohydrate roller-coaster ride that is making you feel "mentally unstable" and addicted to sugar. Relief should come on the first day of the diet and get better as you practice the principles throughout your life. You should also discuss The Fat Burning Diet with your doctor before making any changes.

Q. Whenever I try to change my diet, I get a lot of criticism from my family and friends at work. When I make a change, everyone seems to suddenly become an expert on what is best for me. I then become confused with all the advice, stop making the positive changes, and revert back to my old eating habits. **How do I avoid the critical, negative comments that seem to come my way every time I make a change in my life—especially a positive change?**

A. The best approach for avoiding criticism while making any changes in your life is to discuss your changes with ABSOLUTELY NO ONE! Don't talk about it; DO IT! Then after 2 to 3 months, try discussing your changes and experiences with someone close to you. If they freak out or get heavy on you with guilt trips and fear tactics—or are not supportive of your changes—drop the discussion with them immediately. Suggest that they not share their negative attitude or fears, and let them be. Your changes are for yourself and no one else. What you do is your own private matter and no one's business unless you allow it to become their business. If, on the other hand, you discuss your changes with friends and they are excited and supportive, then keep talking to them! Find your positive supporters, and *spend time with them. You may find yourself with a whole new set of friends, which is exactly what happened in my life.*

Many people will experience fear as they watch YOU take charge of your life, and they may talk negatively about you and the changes you are making. They may try to scare you with cholesterol fear, fat fear, starvation fear, going-against-the-grain fear, and more. As your body fat levels plunge to normal or an athletic low level, many people may even try to scare you into thinking you are "wasting away!" Well, fear not for "there is nothing to fear but fear itself." Also, put your trust in the Lord, and you will be unshakable!

> "The Lord is on my side; I have no fear."
> —Psalm 118:6

Q. I have two children—ages seven and nine. They both cringe at the thought of eating natural foods. *Can they follow The Fat Burning Diet Plan, and how can I get them to stick with it?*

A. *Children ages 2 through 18 do fabulous on The Fat Burning Diet principles if they have a tendency to be overweight. For children of normal weight, it is best to include carbohydrates and starches each day, but use only whole food starches—such as potatoes, yams, whole grains, squash, and brown rice. Eliminate all refined carbohydrates—such as sugar, fructose, corn syrup, sodas, candy bars, desserts, ice cream, white bread, pizza, white pasta, enriched macaroni noodles, and white rice. Serve natural hormone-free meats and eggs, along with plenty of salads, steamed vegetables, nuts, seeds, and fruit. If they are overweight, then utilize low-carb meals every other day when possible. If their weight is normal and they are active, more natural carbohydrates can be consumed, as desired.*

Many parents tell me their children refuse to eat wholesome foods. I always tell them that their children are not really hungry. Have them miss a meal, and give them no junky snacks. Then watch them belly up to the dinner table, begging for your "wholesome" foods. If a child is not hungry at a meal for real food, then he or she should never be forced to eat. Usually a loss of appetite for a child means they ate sugary or high-carbohydrate snacks within 1 to 2 hours before the meal. Take away the junk, and limit snacks to only sliced vegetables or fresh fruit, and your child should suddenly develop a new zest for natural foods.

Q. I am skinny and wish to gain weight. Will The Fat Burning Diet help me accomplish this, or will I lose weight on this program and become even skinnier than I am now?

A. The Fat Burning Diet is actually a weight-normalizing program that allows you to access fat as an energy source approximately 50% of the time. If you are overweight (fat), you will lose fat. If you are underweight (low in muscle tissue), you will gain muscle. By offering your body balanced meals, as The Fat Burning Diet does, you will naturally return to a normal weight that is ideal for you. The secret to gaining weight is to simply increase your daily calorie intake. To gain weight, you can also try eating high-carb moderate-protein meals for three consecutive days, followed by one day of low-carb meals, then repeat the cycle.

Q. I have a sweet tooth and often use artificial sweeteners—such as Equal®, Nutrasweet®, and Sweet-N-Low®. Are these non-nutritive sweeteners okay to use on The Fat Burning Diet?

A. Because of possible negative side effects, I do not advocate the use of any of the artificial sweeteners mentioned above. When you initially begin The Fat Burning Diet, you may desire to use artificial sweeteners because your mind still remembers "sweets." When something natural that you are eating needs to be lightly sweetened, try using a natural herb called "stevia."

Stevia, which is available as a granulated powder, is a natural herb that has a sweet taste. This herb is not classed as a sweetener by the FDA, but it has a delightful sweet taste when mixed with citrus fruits, lemons, limes, strawberries, yogurt, baked goods, protein drinks containing berries, and a variety of other foods. To the best of my knowledge, Jay Robb Enterprises was the first company in America to utilize the herb stevia in a protein powder formula.

Q. I have problems with willpower. I'm easily motivated to change my diet and become healthy, but after a few weeks, I begin to cheat and soon return to my old habits. How do you stay perpetually motivated to always eat properly and be healthy? I want to know your secret!

A. I am no different than you or anyone else on this planet. Changing my diet and lifestyle has been just as challenging for me as the next guy. I have an addictive personality and have had to overcome an extremely strong addiction to carbohy-drates—especially pancakes, pizza, ice cream, and cherry cheesecake. How did I do it? It was easy. I let go and let God sit in the driver's seat. And that, my friend, has made all the dif-ference in the world. (See Chapter 4 for more details.)

If you are feeling defeated, overwhelmed, depressed, fearful, anxiety ridden, and/or lack confidence and motivation in your life, then let go of the "wheel," and let God drive. He knows where He wants you to go in this life because He has a plan for you. He wants to give you a new life. He wants you to be in the best shape possible so He can utilize your body to do His work here on earth.

As long as you hold onto the wheel, you will have problems because there are too many temptations in life. I thought I could do it on my own, but I obviously couldn't. On my own I drove into the ditch every time I saw a cherry cheesecake, a cold beer, a pizza, or a dish of ice cream. I called this driving detour my "addiction ditch," and I swear I spent more time in that ditch than on the road of life—as long as I was the one driving.

Let go of the controls, and let the Lord do all the driving. You have nothing to lose but all your problems, excess weight, and addictions. It's easy to let go. Just pray every day, and don't ever stop. Then trust Him with everything you have, and let go. It's that easy. Ask and you shall receive.

"Freedom from the desire for an answer is essential to the understanding of a problem."
—Krishnamurti

"Pride is the real terrorist of the world."
—The Author

Final Words of Encouragement

"The future is so bright—if I were to look
back, even for a moment, I would be blinded
by darkness instead of guided by the light."
—The Author

My fat burning journey began in 1978 and will continue as long
as the Lord chooses to work through me to share His message.
This journey, which is also now *your* journey, requires patience,
understanding, and never-ending faith.

To ensure success, pray as often as possible for the support
you need to stay on target. Prayer and faith in God are truly my
two secrets to success. Keep in mind that true *success* is a
lifetime journey and commitment, not a goal or destination.

This diet can be your ticket to better health, a better body, and
a better life. The Fat Burning Diet was a gift to me, and now I
am passing it on to you—with only one request. Please share
the information in this book with at least ONE other person.
That's all I ask.

On the following page, I will close with a prayer and inspirational
passage from scripture:

"Dear God,

Thank You for being the beacon of light that allows us to see the truth at all times. Your truth sets us free.

I pray this book will inspire each reader to follow its simple, yet powerful, principles so they can achieve the healthy, harmonious, and balanced life that You have planned for them."

> My thoughts are not your thoughts.
> Nor are My ways your ways—declares the Lord.
> But as the heavens are high above the earth,
> So are My ways above your ways
> And My plans above your plans.
> —Isaiah 55:8-9

His will, His way...all the way,

Jay Robb

Bibliography

Addolorato G, Parente A, de Lorenzi G, et al. 2003. Rapid Regression of Psoriasis in a Coeliac Patient After Gluten-Free Diet: A Case Report and Review of the Literature. *Digestion* 68:9-12.

Albert CM, et al. 2002. Blood Levels of Long-Chain n-3 Fatty Acids and the Risk of Sudden Death. *New England Journal of Medicine* 346:1113-1118.

Beauschesne-Rondeau E, Gascon A, et al. 2003. Plasma Lipids and Lipoproteins in Hypercholesterolemic Men Fed a Lipid-Lowering Diet Containing Lean Beef, Lean Fish, or Poultry. *Am J Clin Nutr.* 77:587-593.

Bengmark S. 2003. Use of Some Pre-, Pro- and Synbiotics in Critically Ill Patients. *Best Pract Res Clin Gastroenterol* 17(5):1-15.

Bosworth HB, Park KS, et al. 2003. The Impact of Religious Practice and Religious Coping on Geriatric Depression. *Int J Geriatr Psychiatry* 18:905-914.

Brand-Miller J, Hayne S, et al. August 2003. Low-Glycemic Index Diets in the Management of Diabetes: A Meta-Analysis of Randomized Controlled Trials. *Diabetes Care* 26(8):2261-2267.

Brichard, SM, Okitolonde W, Henquin. 1988. JCL: Long-Term Improvement of Glucose Homeostasis by Vanadate Treatment in Diabetic Rats. *Endocrinology* 123: 2048-2053.

Bushara KO, Nance M, Gomez CM. January 2004. Antigliadin Antibodies in Huntington's Disease. *Neurology* 62(1 of 2):132-133.

Cahill G, Aoki TT. 1970. *Medical Times* 98.

Collgan, M.D., M. 1993. *Optimum Sports Nutrition.* Advanced Research Press 146-151.

Colev M, Engel H, Mayers M, et al. January-February 2004. Vegan Diet and Vitamin A Deficiency. *Clin Pediatr.* 43:107-109.

Crook, M.D., WG. 1991. *The Yeast Connection.* Professional Books 2-3.

DiPasquale, M.D., M. 1995. *The Anabolic Diet.* Optimum Training Systems 3.

The Fat Burning Diet

Dunstan DW, DeCourten M, Daly RM, et al. 2002. High-Intensity Resistance Training Improves Glycemic Control in Older Patients with Type 2 Diabetes. *Diabetes Care* 25:1729-1736.

Edwards AJ, Vinyard BT, et al. 2003. Consumption of Watermelon Juice Increases Plasma Concentrations of Lycopene and B-Carotene in Humans. *J Nutr.* 133:1043-1050.

Erasmus, U. 1990. *Fats that Heal—Fats that Kill.* Alive Books.

Erasmus, U. 1986. *Fats and Oils.* Alive Books 270.

Elllis, Ph.D., GS. March 1991. *Control of Food to Make Energy.*

Farnsworth E, Luscombe ND, Noakes M, et al. 2003. Effect of a High-Protein, Energy-Restricted Diet on Body Composition, Glycemic Control, and Lipid Concentrations in Overweight and Obese Hyperinsulinemic Men and Women. *Am J Clin Nutr.* 78:31-39.

Fiocchi A, Martelli A, et al. July 2003. Primary Dietary Prevention of Food Allergy. *An Allergy Asthma Immunol.* 91:3-13.

Forman, Ph.D., Robert. 1977. *How to Control Your Allergies.* Larchmont Books 186.

Frei B. July 16, 2003. To C or Not to C, That Is the Question! *J Am Coll Cardiol.* 42(2):253-2.

Giray B, Hincal F, et al. 2001. Status of Selenium and Antioxidant Enzymes of Goitrous Children Is Lower than Healthy Controls and Nongoitrous Children with High Iodine Deficiency. *Biol Trace Elem Res.* 82:35-52.

Gray, R. 1983. *The Colon Health Handbook.* Rockridge Publishing Co. 17.

Hu, FB, et al. 2002. Fish and Omega-3 Fatty Acid Intake and Risk of Coronary Heart Disease in Women. *JAMA* 287:1815-1821.

Hu FB, Cho E, et al. April 15, 2003. Fish and Long-Chain Omega-3 Fatty Acid Intake and Risk of Coronary Heart Disease and Total Mortality in Diabetic Women. *Circulation* 107:1852-1857.

Igram, M.D., C. 1989. *Eat Right or Die Young.* Literary Visions Inc. 68-69.

Ivy JL, Goforth, Jr., HW, et al. 2002. Early Postexercise Muscle Glycogen Recovery Is Enhanced with a Carbohydrate-Protein Supplement. *J Appl Physiol.* 93:1337-1344.

Jensen, D.C., B. 1981. *Tissue Cleansing through Bowel Management.* Jensen 74-75.

Johnston, I. and J. 1990. *Flaxseed (Linseed) Oil and the Power of Omega-3.* Keats Publishing 23.

Kiessling G, Schneider J, Jahreis G. 2002. Long-Term Consumption of Fermented Dairy Products Over 6 Months Increases HDL Cholesterol. *Eur J Clin Nutr.* 56:843-849.

Kime, M.D., ZR. 1980. *Sunlight Could Save Your Life.* World Health Publications 221.

Kirschmann J. 1979. *Nutrition Almanac.* McGraw Hill 144.

Kris-Etherton PM, Harris WS, Appel LJ. November 19, 2002. Fish Consumption, Fish Oil, Omega-3 Fatty Acids, and Cardiovascular Disease. *Circulation* 106:2747-2757.

Kris-Etherton PM, Harris WS, et al. February 2003. Omega-3 Fatty Acids and Cardiovascular Disease: New Recommendations from the American Heart Association. *Arterioscler Thromb Vasc Biol.* 23:151-152.

Layman DK, Boileau RA, et al. 2003. A Reduced Ratio of Dietary Carbohydrate to Protein Improves Body Composition and Blood Lipid Profiles During Weight Loss in Adult Women. *J Nutr.* 133:411-417.

Linskens RK, Huijsdens XW, et al. 2001. The Bacterial Flora in Inflammatory Bowel Disease: Current Insights in Pathogenesis and the Influence of Antibiotics and Probiotics. *Scand J Gastroenterol.* 36(Suppl 234):29-40.

Lundin KEA, Nilsen EM, Scott HG, et al. 2003. Oats Induced Villous Atrophy in Coeliac Disease. *Gut* 52:1649-1652.

McNamara D. May 15, 2003. Regular Breakfast Eaters at Lower Risk for Obesity. *Family Practice News* 10.

McNamara D. July 2003. Vitamin C Derivative Cleared More Acne than Clindamycin 1%. *Skin and Allergy News* 36.

Maffetone, M.D., P. 1993. Eat Fat and Get Fast! *PR Nutrition.*

Marchioli, M.D., Roberto, et al. 2002. Early Protection Against Sudden Death by N-3 Polyunsaturated Fatty Acids After Myocardial Infarction. *Circulation* 105:1897-1903.

Maynard M, Gunnell D, et al. 2003. Fruit, Vegetables, and Antioxidants in Childhood and Risk of Adult Cancer: The Boyd Orr Cohort. *J Epidemiol Community Health* 57:218-225.

Mrdjenovic G, Levitsky DA. June 2003. Nutritional and Energetic Consequences of Sweetened Drink Consumption in 6- to 13-Year-Old Children. *J Pediatr.* 142:604-610.

Nelsen DA. December 15, 2002. Gluten-Sensitive Enteropathy (Celiac Disease): More Common than You Think. *Am Fam Physician* 66(12):2259-2266, 2269-2270.

Nelson KM, Reiber G, Boyko EJ. October 2002. Diet and Exercise Among Adults with Type 2 Diabetes: Findings from the Third National Health and Nutrition Examination Survey (NHANES III). *Diabetes Care* 25(10):1722-1728.

Nieuwenhuizen WF, Pieters RHH, et al. June 21, 2003. Is Candida Albicans a Trigger in the Onset of Coeliac Disease? *Lancet.* 361:2152-2154.

Oeveren, D.C., KV. 1995. *The Nutritional Notebook.*

The Fat Burning Diet

Passwater, Ph.D., R.A. 1993. *The Longevity Factor, Chromium Picolinate*. Keats Publishing 42-43.

Pereira MA, Liu S. 2003. Types of Carbohydrates and Risk of Cardiovascular Disease. *J Women's Health* 12(2):115-122.

Plaskett LG. September 2003. On the Essentiality of Dietary Carbohydrate. *J Nutr Environ Med.* 13(3):161-168.

Rallidis LS, Paschos G, et al. 2003. Dietary Alpha Linolenic Acid Decreases C-Reactive Protein, Serum Amyloid A and Interleukin-6 in Dyslipidaemic Patients. *Atherosclerosis* 167:237-242.

Ramanadham, S, Mongold, JJ, Brwonsey RW, Cros GH, McNeill JH. 1987. Oral Vanadyl Sulfate in the Treatment of Diabetes Mellitus in the Rat. *Am J Physiol.* 257: H904-H911.

Rand WM, Pellett PL, Young VR. 2003. Meta-Analysis of Nitrogen Balance Studies for Estimating Protein Requirements in Healthy Adults. *Am J Clin Nutr* 77:109-127.

Rosenberg, Dr. H. 1974. *The Book of Vitamin Therapy*. Berkley Windhover Books 114-115.

Sabate J. 2003. Nut Consumption and Body Weight. *Am J Clin Nutri.* 78(Suppl):647S-650S.

Santillo B.S., M.H., H. 1987. *Food Enzymes, The Missing Link to Radiant Health*. Hohm Press 2.

Schulze MB, Manson JE, et al. 2003. Processed Meat Intake and Incidence of Type 2 Diabetes in Younger and Middle-Aged Women. *Diabetologia* 46:1465-1473.

Seccareccia F, Alberti-Fidanza A, et al. Vegetable Intake and Long-Term Survival Among Middle-Aged Men in Italy. *Ann. Epidemiol* 13(6):424-430.

Segal E, Dvorkin L, Lavy A, et al. 2003. Bone Density in Axial and Appendicular Skeleton in Patients with Lactose Intolerance: Influence of Calcium Intake and Vitamin D Status. *J Am Coll Nutr.* 22(3):201-207.

South, M.A., J. July 1989. *Optimal Nutrition Review*. Vol. 1, No. 1.

Suga A, Hirano T, Kageyama H, Osaka T, Namba Y, Tsuji M, Miura M, Adachi M, Inoue S. April 2000. Effects of Fructose and Glucose on Plasma Leptin, Insulin, and Insulin Resistance in Lean and VMH-Lesioned Obese Rats. *Am J Physiol Endocrinol Metab* 278(4):E677-E683.

Tamayo C, Richardson MA. May/June 2003. Vitamin C as a Cancer Treatment: State of the Science and Recommendations for Research. *Altern Ther.* 9(3):94-102.

Trebble TM, Wootton SA, et al. 2003. Prostaglandin E2 Production and T Cell Function After Fish-Oil Supplementation: Response to Antioxidant Cosupplementation. *Am J Clin Nutr.* 78:376-382.

Truswell AS. 2002. Meat Consumption and Cancer of the Large Bowel. *Eur J Clin Nutr* 56(Suppl 1):S19-S24.

Waring WS, Goudsmit J, Marwick J, et al. November 2003. Acute Caffeine Intake Influences Central More than Peripheral Blood Pressure in Young Adults. *Am J Hypertens* 16(11 part 1):919-924.

Weaver CM, Boushey CJ. December 2003. Milk - Good for Bones, Good for Reducing Childhood Obesity? *J Am Diet Assoc* 103(12):1598-1599.

Webster, D. 1995. *Achieve Maximum Health: Colon Flora-The Missing Link in Immunity, Health & Longevity.* Hygeia Publishing.

Wien MA, Sabate JM, Ikle DN, et al. 2003. Almonds Vs. Complex Carbohydrates in a Weight Reduction Program. *Int J Obes* 27:1365-1372.

Wilson, M.D., ED. 1993. *Wilson's Syndrome.* Cornerstone Publishing Company 119-123.

Wurtman, J.J., Ph.D. 1986. *Managing Your Mind and Mood through Food.* Rawson Associates 21-23.

Wurtman RJ, Wurtman JJ, et al. 2003. Effects of Normal Meals Rich in Carbohydrates or Proteins on Plasma Tryptophan and Tyrosine Ratios. *Am J Clin Nutr.* 77:128-132.

Yang EJ, Chung HK, et al. 2002. Carbohydrate Intake Is Associated with Diet Quality and Risk Factors for Cardiovascular Disease in U.S. Adults: NHANES III. *J Am Coll Nutr.* 22(1):71-79.

Yessis, M., Ph.D. November 1993. Performance Shorts. *Muscle and Fitness* 35.

Zoler ML. January 15, 2003. Heart Association Advocates Fish Oil Supplements. *Family Practice News* 6.

"I pretty much try to stay in a constant state of confusion just because of the expression it leaves on my face."
—Johnny Depp

Other Popular Works by
Jay Robb

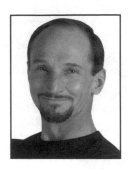

The Fat Burning Diet Cook Book
> (Over 150 mouth-watering fat burning recipes!)

Secrets to Staying Slim (CD)
> (Lose excess fat like never before!)

Successful Bodybuilding Without Steroids (Book)
> (Gain lean muscle mass *without* drugs!)

Ultimate Abdominals in 30 Days (Book)
> (Jay's easy way to a flat stomach!)

Jay Robb's FREE Health-E-newsletter
> (Stay on the cutting-edge of health and fat loss!)

Fit for Christ (Book - Coming Spring 2005)
> (How to stay spiritually fit & connected with God!)

For more information:

1.877.JAY.ROBB / www.JayRobb.com

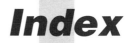

Index

A

B

dry skin, 163, 167

E

egg white protein, 222, 226
Eicosapentaenoic Acid, 164
endurance athlete, 28
enzymes, 153, 154
erythritol, 225
essential fatty acids, 29
excessive exercise, 155
exercise, 32, 33, 34, 35, 43, 147, 148, 149, 150, 151

F

faith, 104
fast food, 129
fat burning, 147, 148, 150, 152
(The) Fat Burning Diet (variations of), 110
fat intake, 37
fat storing hormone, 26
fatigue, 27, 28, 41, 42
fear, 104
feeding the family, 117
fish oil capsules, 165, 166, 220, 232
fitness, 147, 148, 149, 150, 151
flax seed, 165, 166, 167
flax seed oil, 220, 229, 230
food combining, 36, 113, 114
foods and ingredients to avoid, 58
fruit, 114

G

gaining muscle, 170
gaining weight, 44
Gamma-Linolenic Acid, 165
gas, 135, 136, 137, 139
GLA, 165
GLP (Glycogen Loading Principle), 32
glucose, 31, 32, 42, 140
gluten, 28, 29
glycogen, 31, 32, 33, 34, 35, 36, 163, 166
glycogen debt, 24
glycogen management, 31, 32
God, 19, 20, 21, 44, 46, 47, 48, 49, 50, 51, 153, 233, 238

organically grown foods, 121
oxygen, 43

P

Palmitic Acid, 166
pasta, 28, 29
permanent weight management, 31
pH test strips, 36, 42
pizza, 135, 136
Power Pudding, 138, 139
prayer, 19, 20, 49, 50, 51
protein, 24, 25, 27, 28, 29, 36, 38, 40, 53, 55, 58
protein bars, 220, 224, 225, 226
protein drink, 165, 167
protein powder, 219, 221, 225
psoriasis, 167

R

Rabbi Yose, 151
ratios of protein to fat to carbohydrate, 38, 53, 55
raw salad, 38
reactive hypoglycemia, 20
restaurants, 40
running, 147, 148, 149, 150, 151

S

salt, 40, 180
saturated fats, 166
serotonin, 28
shredded, 169
snacking, 37, 39
snacks, 31, 37, 114
sodium chloride, 40
soy protein, 222, 226
starches, 37
Stearic Acid, 165
steroids, 170, 172, 175, 180
stevia, 38, 39, 40, 66, 68, 69, 71, 73, 75, 76, 77, 79, 80, 81, 82, 84, 85, 86, 87, 89, 90, 91, 92, 94, 96, 97, 98, 100, 101, 173, 176, 177, 178, 220, 227
stress, 154, 155, 157, 158, 159, 161
success at dieting, 47
Successful Bodybuilding Without Steroids, 151

X

xylitol, 226

Y

yeast infection, 135
yogurt, 37, 39, 40